# 3D Printing PPE In the Age of COVID-19

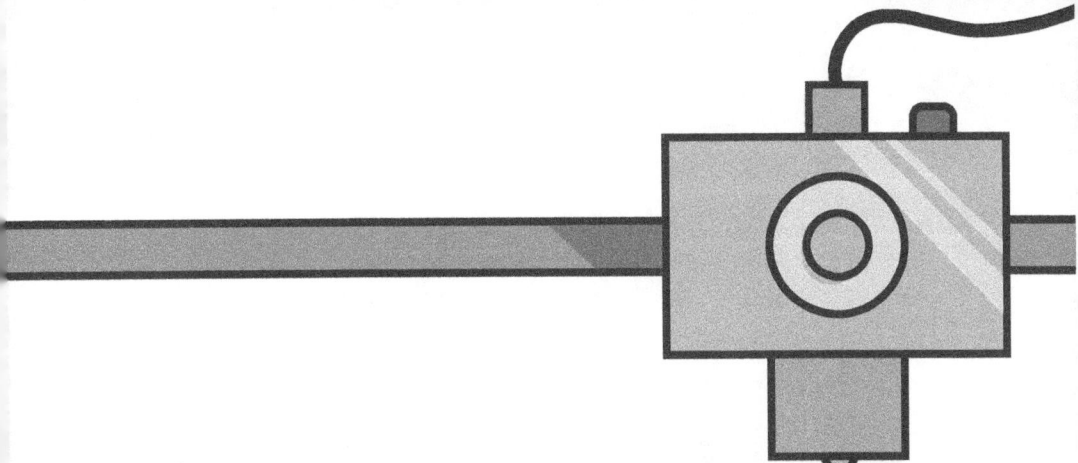

# 3D PRINTING PPE

## IN THE AGE OF COVID-19

Austin Mardon

Olsen Chan, Armita Yousefi, Maisha Fahmida,
Anushka Hasija
and
Catherine Mardon

**GM** PRESS

2020

First Printing: 2020

ISBN: 978-1-77369-183-1

Golden Meteorite Press
103 11919 82 St NW
Edmonton, AB T5B 2W3
www.goldenmeteoritepress.com

We acknowledge the support of Canada Service Corps, TakingITGlobal and the Government of Canada in promotional materials associated with the Project.
Thank you

# CONTENTS

# **Chapter 1**

## INTRODUCTION

With the arrival of Tuesday, December 31st, 2019, crowds and celebrations were seen throughout the world as the day had marked the end of another decade. Filled with feelings of hope and excitement, many people had anticipated the return of the Roaring Twenties. However, unbeknownst to much of the world, the new decade would not be the start of a prosperous period, but the beginning of an international crisis known as the COVID-19 pandemic. This downward spiral first began on New Year's Eve, with the report of a cluster of pneumonia cases in Wuhan, China (World Health Organization [WHO], 2020g). The culprit was soon identified as a novel coronavirus and it was determined to have a large genetic similarity to severe acute respiratory syndrome (SARS) coronavirus (SARS-CoV), the virus responsible for the SARS outbreak of 2003 (Center of Disease Control and Prevention [CDC], 2004; Lu et al., 2020). Due to this finding, the WHO had later announced that the name of the virus will be SARS-CoV-2 and that the disease will be known as COVID-19 (WHO, 2020b). However, unlike SARS-CoV, SARS-CoV-2 is a far more transmissible and infectious virus (Petersen et al., 2020). When this is paired with a long incubation period of 2-14 days, which is the time between an individual's exposure to the virus to the onset of symptoms, it became clear to many experts that this virus is a serious threat to public health and that it held pandemic potential (Adelman et al., 2020). Despite this knowledge, however, many countries had found themselves unprepared and caught off guard as they had underestimated the severity of the rapidly escalating crisis of the COVID-19 pandemic. This is clearly demonstrated by the global depletion personal protective equipment (PPE).

With PPEs often being regarded as the "last line of defence", maintaining a steady supply of PPE is crucial in protecting the very people that risk their lives every day to treat others (Bensadoun, 2020). These PPEs include gloves, gowns, surgical masks, N95 respirators, face shields, and goggles, among many others (Bensadoun, 2020). However, with a rapidly growing number of patients being admitted into hospitals for COVID-19, the demand for PPE has skyrocketed across the globe. Since the ideal situation would be for healthcare professionals to dispose of their PPE between each patient, this could potentially translate to 20 or more masks being used on an average shift (Bensadoun, 2020). With such a large consumption of PPE, it is not difficult to imagine that many governments have struggled to procure a sufficient supply. Although there have been several efforts to increase the domestic production of PPE, the WHO had reported in March that the worldwide manufacturing of PPE needed to increase by 40 per cent in order to meet the global demand (WHO, 2020c). Unfortunately, the process of adjusting production lines and increasing the manufacturing of PPE is considerably time consuming. This presents an urgent issue for various medical facilities as the supply of PPE has already been drained to dangerously low levels. Therefore, without a fast response to the PPE crisis, it is possible that the supply of PPE could be completely depleted before production is increased to sufficient levels.

To many, this would be an unacceptable and heartbreaking scenario as many healthcare professionals have already been enduring dangerous and unfortunate conditions. Dr. Calvin Sun, an emergentologist in New York City, has been witnessing and experiencing these horrors firsthand (James, 2020). While documenting his experiences in April, he reported that some emergency rooms throughout the city had already run out of gowns and N95 respirators (James, 2020). With the PPE shortage reaching such severe levels, he had been forced to improvise and create his own makeshift PPE (James, 2020). Though it is far from state-of-the-art equipment, he attends work each day wearing his ski goggles and ski jacket (James, 2020). Despite these demoralizing conditions, many healthcare professionals, including Dr. Sun, have continued to go to work and put themselves at risk in hopes of saving another patient (James, 2020). While these conditions alone are already an unimaginable sacrifice, many of the frontline workers have also been forced to put aside their family and personal lives. Dr. Rachel Patzer, an associate professor at

Emory University School of Medicine, has described how this virus has had an impact on her family (O'Kane, 2020). Since her husband is an emergency room doctor that has been actively treating COVID-19 patients, the couple has felt no choice, but to have the husband isolate himself in their garage apartment, away from his family and 3-week-old newborn (O'Kane, 2020). Although this is the best course of action to prevent their family from becoming infected by the virus, Dr. Patzer cannot help but think about the amount of time that her husband will be away from their family (O'Kane, 2020). Every week that he spends in the garage apartment is another week that he is unable to hold his newborn child. With infancy being such an important period for developing bonds of love and trust, it is truly agonizing to hear that a doctor believes that they must sacrifice this valuable and limited time to protect those that he loves from potentially being exposed to the virus (CDC, n.d.).

As it is clear from these anecdotes, the frontline workers have been regularly experiencing horrendous conditions and yet, many of them have been continually putting themselves at risk to help treat others. These acts of altruism are truly admirable, and patients are incredibly fortunate that there are members of their community that are willing to put their own lives at risk to save those in need. To demonstrate their gratitude, many eager and determined individuals have been examining various ways to help address the PPE crisis. One such method has been explored by companies, academic institutions, and eager individuals as they have volunteered their own time and resources to 3D print PPE for donation (Thompson, 2020). Since 3D printable PPE designs can be easily accessed online, those who own 3D printers are capable of beginning the manufacturing process immediately after download (Clifton et al., 2020). This unique advantage allows for a rapid response, one that is arguably faster than traditional methods. As previously mentioned, speed is absolutely crucial during this pandemic as there is a large immediate need for PPE. Thus, the use of 3D printers may be used to buy some additional time and prevent the complete depletion of PPE. With such a monumental impact on our healthcare system, it is crucial to understand what 3D printing is and what this technology truly entails.

With numerous news reports praising volunteers for manufacturing and donating 3D printed PPE to local medical facilities, many people have been conditioned to believe that this event is extremely beneficial, and that 3D printing is the solution to the shortage crisis (Thompson, 2020). Although it is true that these noble and philanthropic actions are worth being praised, it is important to understand that 3D printing is not perfect. As with all technology, there are various drawbacks, concerns and negative implications that are associated with this technology. For this reason, it is crucial to have a thorough understanding of additive manufacturing before supporting or opposing its widespread use during this pandemic. This would include a variety of topics, such as how additive manufacturing works, in which aspects is it superior or inferior to other manufacturing techniques, what the potential applications of this technology are, what the positive and negative implications are, and which situations 3D printing is being used for. By exploring these different topics, people would be able to develop an independent and informed opinion about 3D printing PPE and decide whether or not the benefits outweigh the cons.

Despite appearing trivial, an opinion on the 3D printing of PPE could potentially have an impact on the future of this technology as an overwhelming amount of support could result in a larger regular presence of additive manufacturing in the medical field. In contrast, those who oppose 3D printing can also have a large impact as further research may be conducted to address their specific concerns and to make additive manufacturing a much more appealing technology. Evidently, regardless of the opinion, the fact that people have a vested interest in the field of 3D printing can potentially lead to significant change and improvements. This may be particularly useful as the knowledge and improvements gained from this experience can be potentially transferred to future situations. Whether it be another viral outbreak or a different disaster where there is a large shortage of desperately needed products, the world would much be better prepared to handle these critical situations by learning from the past and making improvements. Thus, by providing a simplified summary of the role of 3D printing PPE during the COVID-19 pandemic, this book hopes to promote an interest in the field and potentially spark further research to improve the application of this technology in the future.

In the following chapter, this book will provide introductory information on the impacts and development of the pandemic, exploring various topics, including the symptoms of COVID-19, the global shortage of PPE, the economic repercussions, and the contrasting situations in different countries around the world. The subsequent chapter will then delve deeper into this topic as it focuses on varying situations and responses of the four most affected countries in terms of the number of confirmed COVID-19 cases. Afterwards, the next chapter will explore the importance of preventative measures, tackling topics such as the modes of transmission and public health measures. By exploring these different topics, one would be able to construct an accurate representation of the ongoing situation and understand the emotions and thought processes of everyone involved. Without a comprehensive understanding of the severity of the situation and the repercussions of an inadequate public health response, it would be difficult to comprehend why the shortage of PPE is such a detrimental crisis. Thus, the purpose of these initial chapters is to establish the context of the situation and explain why this dire issue needs to be addressed as soon as it possibly can.

Following the illustration of this urgent problem, the subsequent two chapters will investigate the proposed solution of 3D printing PPE. Beginning with its history, this chapter aims to provide insight into the dynamic nature of additive manufacturing. Since its conception, interest in this technology has dramatically increased through the past several decades and with a plethora of innovators harnessing this technology in the field of medicine. With the potential to manufacture a wide range of products, it is clear that 3D printing is not limited to PPEs. Even outside of the context of COVID-19 it is evident that the technology of additive manufacturing is monumental. Thus, the next two chapters will examine the various methods of 3D printing to provide a more detailed understanding of this innovative technology. This includes the 3D printing methods of stereolithography (SLA), selective laser sintering (SLS) and fused deposition modeling (FDM), and polymer jet fabrication. Once this understanding is achieved, the subsequent chapters will explore alternative forms of manufacturing, including injection molding, stamping, and hydroforming. The purpose of these chapters is to allow for a comparison between these manufacturing techniques and 3D printing. This would highlight the unique advantages and disadvantages of 3D printing as well as provide an understanding of how these manufacturing techniques may be used in combination to create a much more effective response.

Afterwards, the following chapters would explore the various forms of PPE, including face masks, N95 respirators, face shields, visors, hazmat suits and gloves. Beginning with the topic of face masks, the chapter will investigate how masks prevent the spread of disease as well as the differences between traditional masks, 3D printed masks and cloth masks. Since 3D printing PPE is not the only approach that is being used, it is important to examine the pros and cons of the alternatives to determine the superior approach. However, it is noteworthy that simply because an approach is inferior does not mean that it has no use. Different approaches can offer different benefits which is why they both need to be investigated thoroughly so that the use of these two approaches can be optimized. Following this examination, the subsequent chapters will provide a general overview of the other PPEs that were previously mentioned by investigating their unique functions, manufacturing regulations, and overall effectiveness. By the end of these chapters, the reader should gain a comprehensive understanding of the role of each PPE and how 3D printing technology may be utilized in its manufacturing. Afterwards, the next chapter will then examine how 3D printing can further improve these PPEs by customizing each product for specific people and settings. Since additive manufacturing is capable of producing these customized products at a relatively low cost, the purpose of this chapter is to investigate the extent of this advantage and explore the limitations of 3D printing with regards to customization (Berman, 2012).

Lastly, the final chapter before the conclusion will explore the drawbacks, concerns, and limitations of 3D printing technology. As previously explained, the purpose of this book is to provide a holistic view of 3D printing and discuss the various strengths and weaknesses of this technology. Since a large portion of the chapters discuss the various applications and advantages of additive manufacturing, an additional section on the concerns and limitations is necessary to counteract the largely positive portrayal of 3D printing. Therefore, discussing these aspects of additive manufacturing may allow for a fairer and less biased assessment of this technology. By the end of the book, it is hoped that the reader would be able to formulate their own opinion on the 3D printing of PPE and possibly even develop a newfound interest in this technology.

# Chapter 2

## COVID-19 CONTEXT

With the COVID-19 pandemic claiming more lives than any other plagues in recent human history, conspiracy theories have spiraled out of control all across the internet. Is the COVID-19 pandemic a message of apocalypse from the omnipotent God? Is it nature's long-awaited revenge on humans? Or is it a man-made virus funded by world powers? Initially, many sources had speculated that the newest strain had originated from a wet market named Huanan Seafood Wholesale Market in Wuhan, where wild animals, seafood and exotic livestock are slaughtered under open-air with little to no hygienic practices. On March 11th, 2020, the World Health Organization officially declared COVID-19 as a pandemic and cleared suspicions of strains of flu or simply another health crisis confined to a specific region of the world (World Health Organization [WHO], 2020g). Indeed, the number of cases soared to the millions while the death counts reached hundreds of thousands (Johns Hopkins Coronavirus Resource Center, 2020). Unfortunately, it will continue to do so until the invention of the long-awaited COVID-19 vaccine. According to the John Hopkins University COVID-19 Map, the map counts about 22,397,881 cases and 786,269 deaths as of August 19, 2020 (Johns Hopkins Coronavirus Resource Center, 2020).

Frequently asked questions about the virus include visible symptoms, the need for hospitalization, community spread, and many more. Perhaps, the answers vary depending on the country of residence and the severity of the virus contamination in the region. In essence, the common symptoms of COVID-19 entail fever, chills, fatigue and dry cough, but the lesser-known symptoms include muscle aches, runny or blocked noses, sore throat, headache, conjunctivitis and loss of smell or taste (CDC, 2020a). To reduce the burden on incoming patients at major hospitals, patients in various countries are told to self-isolate at home as about 80% of patients are able to recover without hospitalization (WHO, 2020d). When there are severe symptoms that impair proper breathing, consciousness and the mobility of the patient, they should seek immediate medical assistance. Fortunately, COVID-19 has a high recovery rate in youths and middle-aged men and women, but the most vulnerable populations include the elderly and those with pre-existing medical conditions (Center of Disease Control and Prevention [CDC], 2020c). These include cancer, chronic kidney disease, asthma, type 1 diabetes, liver disease, and hypertension according to the CDC (2020c). Droplets of cough, also known as respiratory droplets, transmit this strain of coronavirus from the nose and mouth (Schwartz & King, 2020). Researchers have been exploring the evolution of the virus and investigating whether it could have possibly become airborne.

Although it is essential for governments to increase the prevalence of testing, the process of testing can be strenuous and burdensome for healthcare workers. Therefore, governments worldwide are encouraging individuals to practice preventative measures to contain the spread as much as possible and limit the number of people who can possibly become infected. In Canada, healthcare professionals advise social distancing (also known as physical distancing) of 2 metres from others, both in indoors and outdoors settings, wearing masks, using hand sanitizer or hand wash for at least 15-20 seconds, and self-isolating from public areas if symptoms of COVID-19 are prominent. In the province of Ontario, the government has requested all citizens to wear masks indoors as of July 18th, 2020 (Government of Canada, 2020a). With community transmission becoming a point of concern in many countries, various parts of the world have begun to mandate the use of masks (Government of Canada, 2020a).

Next, with the topic of herd immunity, 'herd' is a term used for the community or groups of people. Some highly populated countries have talked about herd immunity as a strategy of slowing the spread. Herd immunity occurs when the spread of a disease significantly slows as a result of a large portion of the population developing immunity to the disease (Mayo Clinic, 2020). It is developed through a vaccine or through acquired antibodies after the majority of the population has contracted and recovered from disease. Despite the infectious nature of COVID-19, developing herd immunity for most of the population can be deemed an effective preventative strategy. Thus, in the United States, over 70% of the population out of 328 million people have to recover from COVID-19 to stop the pandemic (Mayo Clinic, 2020). Further research has yet to be conducted about the possible implications between second-time coronavirus infections and herd immunity.

Herd immunity or not, physical protection with masks, gloves, face shields and other examples of PPE have become the new norm for not only healthcare professionals and frontline workers, but for the general public as well. To emphasize, the World Health Organization asks for the maintenance of hand and respiratory hygiene as well as the daily usage of masks by both caregivers and patients (WHO, 2020h). At the start of the pandemic, anxious residents hoarded essential supplies, disinfectants, and protective equipment, thereby leading to a shortage that has negatively impacted other citizens and hospital staff. Similarly, certain governments around the world have also demonstrated a similar response to the pandemic as they have begun limiting their exports of PPE. This was seen in the beginning of April as the company 3M was stopped from delivering millions of N95 masks to Canada and Latin America by the White House (The Canadian Press, 2020). With these PPEs providing the best protective barrier against COVID-19, this was seen as an act of betrayal and shock to many Canadians (The Canadian Press, 2020). Whether it is hoarding essential supplies in the grocery store or banning the delivery of essential protective equipment, the phrase "the survival of the fittest" describes the complexity of human nature and diplomacy. Due to the ever-exceeding need of protective equipment, regional, national and international companies in all disciplines have begun manufacturing the needed equipment for essential services and public with great innovation. While some small businesses sewed masks for frontline workers, bigger companies used modern machinery for the mass production of protective gear (The Canadian Press, 2020). Moreover, tech companies have also developed innovative designs for 3D printing masks and other personal protective equipment for the post-pandemic era. The initiative of 3D printing personal protective equipment can prevent the shortages of supplies while also saving time and money. Perhaps a more positive aspect amidst such unprecedented times is the efforts of communities to support the frontlines workers.

In Canada, the COVID-19 pandemic has led to significant change in the family and work life of Canadians. The new normal consisted of working from home, wearing masks in grocery stores, having children attend online school and keeping public spaces closed until quarantine restrictions were lifted. During this time, the excessive use of technology among teens and children has peaked to an all-time high. The social aspects of people's lives were significantly affected as many people were no longer able to have family dinners, friends meet-ups, or any social gatherings in general. As a consequence, this pandemic has proved to be an especially excruciating time for those with various psychological disorders, such as depression, loneliness, anxiety and many other types of mental disorders. Additionally, domestic violence has also reportedly been a rising issue among many households, and many non-profit organizations have been granting shelter and aid for victims (Zhu et al., 2020). However, the effects of this pandemic are not solely confined to the walls of each household as many communities have been affected as a whole. This is clearly displayed in Canada as the country has failed to see the colours, traditions, festivals and cultural gatherings of this diverse nation as it attempts to prevent the transmission of coronavirus. With community being such an important aspect of social and family lives, being unable to access the resources, people and events that we have come to love makes us wonder what human life was like before.

While the social implications are manageable, the economic fall is far worse. With the combination of the debt accumulated from government relief and COVID-19 related initiatives, and the contraction of the Gross Domestic Product (GDP) as a result of the strict lockdown order, it is projected that the Canadian economy shrank by more than 8.6 percent, a larger change than the financial hit of the recession in 2008 and 2009 (Evans, 2020). This is worsened by the fact that the increased rate of unemployment prevents consumers from fueling the economy and spending money, thereby revealing another indication of an economic recession (Evans, 2020). In the long run, this could translate to increased taxes and reduced social programs and benefits for low income families, vulnerable groups and students. However, on the bright side, Canada has consistently demonstrated a low debt-to-GDP ratio, meaning that Canada will have a better chance to recover and pay back its debts (Evans, 2020).

From a scientific perspective, the development of vaccines and COVID-19 related research has surpassed the expectations of many people. With the recently acquired emergency government funding, many universities and hospitals have used these funds to study more about SARS-CoV-2, identify possible courses of treatment and enhance vaccine development. While it is true that healthcare professionals and frontline workers have been some of Canada's most remarkable heroes, it is important to recognize the courageous efforts made by the other essential workers. Whether they work in grocery stores, essential services, or the healthcare industry, they are all worthy of praise. Various news outlets and social media platforms have always highlighted the collective impact of these heroes and have showcased their sacrifices to help millions of people. From restaurants providing free meals to volunteering initiatives that take care of people's children, the community wide effort to support frontline workers is absolutely remarkable. Without this collective effort, overcoming and flattening the curve of infection rates would not have been possible.

Unfortunately, during this fight against the COVID-19 pandemic, thousands of healthcare professionals, including doctors, nurses and technicians, have passed away as a result of treating COVID-19 patients. Lack of PPE and the fear of transmitting COVID-19, it is understandable that the healthcare professionals are subject to significant fatigue and stress (Gan et al., 2020). To worsen their seemingly poor conditions, doctors are also often faced with ethical and legal dilemmas of whether or not to treat patients on ventilators. With widespread shortages of medical equipment and PPE, doctors are frequently forced to decide whether they should prioritize their limited resources elsewhere (Remuzzi & Remuzzi, 2020). In another study with a sample size of 5062 healthcare workers, women and workers with chronic diseases and psychological disorders were found to be more prone to anxiety, depression and stress during this pandemic (Zhu et al., 2020). With many doctors living with young children, elders and family members with underlying health conditions, the fear of potentially spreading COVID-19 to their loved ones can potentially increase the frequency of anxiety and stress disorders for healthcare workers (Zhu et al., 2020). A case in point is the untimely death of an emergency doctor from an infected COVID-19 patient, alongside 14 frontline workers being infected (Schwartz & King, 2020). While many healthcare professionals have isolated themselves from their families as a safety precaution, the implications of such actions may develop into loneliness and depression if this pandemic prolongs.

Many countries around the world have taken severe measures to stop the spread of COVID-19. While the virus itself does not directly discriminate against the residents of developing or developed countries, there is a visible correlation between the social measures, size, population, financial aid, and relief packages and the recovery rates among the developed and developing countries (Remuzzi & Remuzzi 2020). Developed countries are able to help residents with strict quarantine procedures, social distancing measures, mass testing, tracing technology, free healthcare and government emergency funds while the infrastructures and economies of many developing countries prevent effective COVID-19 responses, such as strict quarantine procedures. Moreover, in many developed nations, such as Canada, citizens have the choice to stay home or work, a luxury that many people around the globe do not have. They also lack the funding or the resources from their government to be able to afford healthcare and receive emergency relief funding. With such limited support from their government, many people are forced to choose between staying at home and potentially starving to death or go to work with the risk of contracting COVID-19. Although the effects of this pandemic reach all corners of the globe, it is important for people of the developed world to recognize their privilege during this unfortunate time.

In wealthy countries, such as Taiwan, governments were able to take precautions immediately and implement COVID-19 contact tracing phone apps to help flatten the curve (Tomazin, 2020). The term 'flattening' or 'lowering' the curve in this context means the reduction of COVID-19 cases to slow the transmission of this disease. This is seen in New Zealand as its small population and government employment and emergency benefits allowed for the quarantining of residents, thereby bringing the number of active cases down to zero (Tomain, 2020). Germany also stayed ahead of the curve by mass-testing more than two million people and they have maintained this policy of large-scale testing as an effort to prevent the resurgence of the second wave (Tomazin, 2020). In Canada, the government has made a large response to address the falling economy and worsening unemployment rates (Government of Canada, 2020a). By dedicating over nine billion dollars to the welfare of individuals, businesses and students, the government hopes to alleviate the economic burden caused by this pandemic as well as promote healthcare research for COVID-19 and other attempts to flatten the curve (Government of Canada, 2020a). According to the World Health Organization, Canada's quarantine measures, universal healthcare, plentiful hospital equipment and widespread testing has helped flatten its curve (Jones, 2020; Tomazin, 2020).

In contrast, various countries such as Venezuela are not nearly as successful at tackling this pandemic as they face extreme equipment and doctors' shortages (Tomazin, 2020). In developing countries such as Bangladesh, the government and healthcare institutions have failed to equip doctors with protective equipment, which led to the demise of many healthcare professionals (Tomazin, 2020). These implications put many of the world's poverty-stricken countries in a continuous battle with COVID-19 due to lack of resources, healthcare and funding. Nonetheless, they can potentially recover if there is a large international effort to support these impoverished people. Through the international aid of masks, ventilators, and medicine by developed countries and through the development of strategies to stop the spread of COVID-19 in large and dense populations, the people in the developing world would have a larger chance at survival and economic recovery.

Although it is clear that the developing world has been heavily hit by this pandemic, it is noteworthy that the United States, India and Brazil are some of the world's most affected nations (Johns Hopkins Coronavirus Resource Center, 2020; Moulson, 2020). While France, Germany and the United Kingdom were able to overcome the first wave of COVID-19, the United States seems to show very slow improvement, despite being a financial and economic world power. From the very beginning, the uncontrollable growth of COVID-19 infections are due to the uncoordinated government led by President Donald Trump, who tweeted for "badge of honour" for being able to handle testing alongside the dysfunctional healthcare system (Sink, 2020). To highlight, the quarantine and lockdown measures are different in each state, as well as the number of residents who are more compliant to follow such strict rules and regulation in the "land of the free/home of the brave" (Sink, 2020). Florida, for instance, has opened up its beaches, amusement parks and restaurants and is planning to open schools despite the rising number of cases every day. With such a large focus on reopening the economy, it has led many to wonder what is the purpose of being a wealthy nation when it can not prevent the deaths and sufferings of its citizens?

Since the official announcement of the pandemic, many countries are starting to reopen with the implementation of various frameworks to minimize the transmission as much as possible (Moulson, 2020). Small businesses, restaurants, parks and non-essential services are the first steps towards reopening the economy and adapting to the new COVID-19 related changes in daily life. Many Canadian provinces and American states are opening in stages to test out safety procedures and social distancing measures in public spaces. In Europe, countries such asGermany, Spain, Italy and the United Kingdom have recently opened some of their education system, job market, and travel and tourism industries as an effort to revitalize the economy (Moulson, 2020). Most leaders have demonstrated that economic prosperity outweighs the risks associated with countries' openings (Moulson, 2020). However, it is key to implement precautionary measures to prevent the possibility of an uncontrolled second wave. With the burdening of country after country with financial debts, health disparities, social and cultural voids, it is clear that COVID-19 has successfully created a legacy that will never be forgotten in human history.

# Chapter 3

## AN INTERNATIONAL REVIEW OF THE SUPPLY OF PPE DURING THE COVID-19 PANDEMIC

Although the spread of the COVID-19 pandemic has reached almost all corners of the Earth, there are significant differences in the government policies and experiences of different countries. To understand the supply of PPE and the situation in different countries around the world, this chapter will investigate these ideas in the four most affected countries with regards to COVID-19 cases. As of July 24th, 2020, these countries, in decreasing order of cases, are the United States, Brazil, Russia, and India (World Health Organization [WHO], 2020j). All of the following numbers and statistics in this chapter will be as of July 24th, 2020 unless specified otherwise.

With over four million confirmed cases, the United States leads both the continent of North America and the rest of the world as the country with the highest number of confirmed COVID-19 cases (Boynton, 2020). The next two North American countries to follow behind the United States are Mexico and Canada with roughly 370,000 and 100,000 cases respectively (WHO, 2020j). With such a massive number of infected patients in the United States, it is understandable that the demand for PPE has exponentially increased since the onset of the pandemic. During the first few months, many of the major hospitals in the U.S. were overwhelmed with patients and they had struggled to meet the increased demand for PPE (Dunn & Fitzpatrick, 2020). Although the situation has improved in these major hospitals, the PPE shortage continues to persist throughout the country in rural health facilities, primary care offices, nursing homes, and prisons, among many other facilities (Wan, 2020).

According to Rear Admiral John Polowczyk, the individual in charge of the White House's supply chain task force, over one-fourth of U.S. states have less than a 30-day supply of PPE remaining. This dwindling supply has left many healthcare providers vulnerable to the virus and forced to reuse PPE. In a survey of over 14,000 nurses from across the country, the American Nurses Association found that 79 percent of nurses were required or encouraged to reuse PPE (Dunn & Fitzpatrick, 2020). This is a major concern as there is a possibility that the nurses would be reusing contaminated PPE, thereby putting both them and their patients at major risk of being infected. Additionally, a New York Times article had also reported that at Memorial City Medical Center in Houston, doctors that had been treating COVID-19 patients had been advised to reuse N95 masks for up to 15 days (Jacobs, 2020). With such poor working conditions, many public health experts and major medical associations have criticized the White House's response. Many of them believe that had the government been more aggressive with procuring and distributing PPE during the early stages of the pandemic, the PPE shortage could have been avoided (Jacobs, 2020). In contrast, White House officials believe that the PPE shortages have been blown out of proportion as they explain that the United States has drastically increased both the manufacturing and stockpile of PPE in most states (Wan, 2020). However, regardless of how the government may have performed in the past several months, the main concern should be how the United States plans to provide adequate amounts of PPE to frontline workers.

As an effort to increase domestic PPE production, President Donald Trump has invoked the Defense Production Act after months of reluctancy (Higgins-Dunn & Kim, 2020). This law, which originated in the 1950s, can be used to compel U.S. companies to begin manufacturing PPE (Higgins-Dunn & Kim, 2020). With this law, the Department of Health and Human Services (HHS) has given contracts to 19 companies to manufacture emergency supplies (Alvarez et al., 2020). This includes 600 million N95 respirators and face masks, but it is reported that only half of the order will be delivered by December 2020 (Alvarez et al., 2020). To ensure an adequate supply of PPE for healthcare workers, the HHS and FEMA, the Federal Emergency Management Agency, have also imported over 102 million N95 masks and 139 million gloves from overseas (Alvarez et al., 2020). However, many states have expressed that this federal supply of PPE has only made up a small portion of their stockpiles and that they have acquired much of their PPE on their own, thus demonstrating the government's inadequacy/shortcomings in targeting these dire shortages (Mulvihill & Fassett, 2020).

In addition to the efforts made by the federal and state governments, the American people have also started helping the cause in a variety of ways. In the past few months, American physicians have created a nonprofit organization known as #GetUsPPE which aims to distribute PPE through donated equipment and funds (Wan, 2020). According to Megan Ranney, the co-founder of #GetUsPPE, this nonprofit was created as a temporary solution to the PPE crisis, but, to her disappointment, nothing has appeared to change as no larger permanent solution has been created (Wan, 2020). Additionally, many Americans have also turned to 3D printing to help support the cause. For instance, in Colorado, over 1500 people have volunteered for the initiative "Make4Covid" which has been 3D printing PPE for healthcare workers (Dwyer & Yoo, 2020). To deliver the PPE to rural areas, volunteers have even begun flying donated planes to transport masks and face shields to remote hospitals (Dwyer & Yoo, 2020). Evidently, despite the criticisms that have surrounded the White House's response to the crisis, it is clear that through the talent and resources of the American people, philanthropic Americans will do whatever they can to support their frontline workers.

In South America, Brazil is leading the continent with the largest number of cases and it currently holds the title of having the second largest number of confirmed COVID-19 cases in the world (WHO, 2020j). Behind Brazil, the next most affected South American countries are Peru, Chile, and Colombia (WHO, 2020j). Similarly to other South American countries, the PPE export restrictions imposed by foreign countries have significantly contributed to the substantial PPE deficit in Brazil (United Nations Economic Commission for Latin America and the Caribbean [UNECLAC], 2020). According to a report from the Economic Commission for Latin America and the Caribbean, the region's supply of PPE, mechanical ventilators, test kits, medicine, and other medical supplies are largely sourced from foreign countries (UNECLAC, 2020; Rubin et al., 2020). With less than four percent of these products being sourced from within the region itself, this leaves Latin American and Caribbean countries, such as Brazil, to be highly dependent on imports (UNECLAC, 2020; Rubin et al., 2020). This has demonstrated severe consequences as four of the top five suppliers in this region have imposed restrictions on their medical exports, thereby resulting in a substantial PPE deficit.

The effects of this shortage are seen clearly in Brazil as roughly 18,000 nurses have been infected with the virus and 182 of them have died from COVID-19 as of June 10 (Rubin et al., 2020). Brazilian doctors have also experienced the effects – Pedro Archer, an ICU doctor and the director of the doctor's union in Rio, expressed that doctors in the public sector use the same PPE all day and that a doctor dies every other day (Walsh, 2020). With such poor working conditions, this has contributed to the growing shortage of healthcare workers and Brazil currently accounts for the largest number of deaths among nurses in the world (Fagundes, 2020). However, it is important to note that the lack of PPE is not the sole reason for these deaths as the poor response and leadership from the government has significantly contributed to the overwhelmingly large number of COVID-19 cases. Many members of the government, including President Jair Bolsonaro, have frequently downplayed the severity of the virus and have undermined public health efforts. Not only has Bolsonaro openly criticized the stay-at-home orders, but he has even attended anti-lockdown protests (Fonseca & Paraguassu, 2020; France-Presse, 2020). With such conflicting responses from the government, it is easy to understand why Brazilian healthcare workers have been overwhelmed by patients.

Despite the mixed responses from most of the Brazilian government, there has been a significant effort made by the Ministry of Health, governors, and other political figures to resolve the PPE crisis. For instance, the Ministry of Health has been working tirelessly to supply Brazilian hospitals with PPE, reportedly sending 14.2 million surgical masks along with many other types of medical supplies and equipment to the most affected regions of Brazil (Scalzaretto, 2020). The former health minister, Luiz Mandetta, has also opposed the President as well as he strongly advocated for citizens to stay at home to prevent the spread of the virus. Furthermore, the former health minister has also encouraged citizens to produce homemade masks as it was announced that the health ministry's reserve for medical supplies had been completely depleted (Farr, 2020; Walen et al., 2020). In addition to the efforts made by the Brazilian government, the Brazilian people, including artisans and university researchers, have also made a considerable effort. In the rural city of Ipiranga, many artisans have begun manufacturing medical masks and hair caps while researchers at the Federal University of Sao Paulo have decided to put their projects aside and use their facility and 3D printing resources to manufacture PPE (United Nations Information Centres Rio, 2020; Scalzaretto, 2020) . Unfortunately, these efforts will not be sufficient in the long run and Brazil will need to increase both its domestic production and imports of PPE. However, with reports that the United States has been outbidding other countries and diverting away medical supplies that were intended for Brazil, the international shortage of PPE has made it increasingly difficult to obtain foreign PPE (Farr, 2020; Willsher et al., 2020; Peel et al., 2020). When this is paired with political opposition from many members of the Brazilian government, it is clear that an effective COVID-19 response in Brazil is a particularly difficult task.

According to the World Health Organization, the European region has reported the second largest number of confirmed COVID-19 cases with the top five most affected countries in decreasing order being: the Russian Federation, the United Kingdom, Spain, Italy, and Turkey (WHO, 2020i). In Russia, there has been a significant deficit of PPE as described by Russian President, Vladimir Putin (Rainsford, 2020). A major contributor to this shortage has been the long and tedious process of ordering PPEs. Previously, hospitals and doctors were unable to directly order PPE; instead, they were required to submit a request to the Department of Health. After a review by the government, the supplies would then be ordered and delivered. Although a new law was implemented to expedite the process, the PPE shortage had already grown to be a serious issue by the time the law was introduced.

During early stages of the PPE shortage in Russia, the Russian government had attempted to silence healthcare professionals and prevent them from voicing their concerns online by criminalizing the spread of "fake news" about the virus (Dyer, 2020). Many medical professionals had also reported that they have been threatened with death or prosecution for raising awareness about the widespread shortages (Elliott, 2020). With healthcare professionals reportedly comprising nearly seven percent of the country's COVID-19 deaths, the lack of PPE has forced many frontline workers to resign (Khurshudyan, 2020). However, the government has made an effort to resolve this crisis as it has significantly increased both the production and imports of PPEs. In one month, Russia had demonstrated a tenfold increase in mask production with 8.5 million masks being produced per day (Rainsford, 2020). During the same time frame, Russia had also drastically increased the production of protective suits as they had gone from producing 3,000 suits per day to 100,000 suits (Rainsford, 2020).

To further assist the PPE crisis in Russia, significant contributions have been made by Russian citizens and NGOs. For instance, Russian billionaire and majority shareholder of Norilsk Nickel, Vladimir Potanin, has donated approximately $13.1 million through his foundation to support nonprofit organizations (Dawkins, 2020). Additionally, Norilsk Nickel has also donated $142 million to assist in the purchasing of medical equipment and PPE for medical institutions (Dawkins, 2020). In addition to these efforts, hundreds of NGOs have also been created or have diverted their attention to aid in the COVID-19 response. One such organization is the Zhivoy Foundation which has directed its efforts to purchase PPEs and deliver them directly to PPE-deprived hospitals (Weir, 2020). However, despite all of these efforts, the PPE shortage in Russia continues to persist and further action is needed to resolve this issue.

In Asia, the heavily populated nation of India has been leading the continent with the largest number of confirmed COVID-19 cases. The South Asian country has reported approximately 1.2 million cases, thereby making it the third most affected country in the world (WHO, 2020j). With such a large number of cases, the demand for PPE has drastically increased. Unfortunately, the Indian government has been struggling to procure the supply of PPE and there is currently a large deficit (Pandey, 2020). According to a BBC article that was published on April 13th, 2020, "India needs at least a million PPE kits, as well as 40 million N95 masks, 20 million surgical masks and a million litres of hand sanitisers at the moment" (Pandey, 2020). These numbers were reported by the government-owned corporation of HLL Lifecare Limited (Pandey, 2020). As a consequence of this large deficit, many medical professionals have contracted the virus themselves and many others have decided to manufacture their own PPE from raincoats and bin bags (Farmer & Wallen, 2020; Sarda, 2020). To raise awareness about these poor working conditions, many healthcare professionals have protested in the streets and spoke out on social media. However, similarly to other countries, such as Russia, many of these medical professionals have also been threatened, arrested, and forced to resign for openly speaking about the PPE shortages (Farmer & Wallen, 2020). According to a Telegraph article, one Indian doctor that had complained about the shortage on Twitter has been arrested for "inciting communal tension and criminal intimidation" (Farmer & Wallen, 2020).

Although the censorship of medical professionals has contributed to the public discontent of the Indian government's response to the crisis, criticism has also stemmed from the slow response during the early months of this pandemic. Public health experts, such as Anant Bhan, have argued that the Indian government could have both started stockpiling PPE and increased production much earlier in the year (Farmer & Wallen, 2020; Pandey, 2020). Since increasing production involves the time-consuming process of procuring raw materials and adjusting production lines, an early response during the first few months of this pandemic could have provided manufacturers with a sufficient amount of time to meet the growing demand for PPE (Farmer & Wallen, 2020; Pandey, 2020). To compensate for this lost time, the federal ministry of health announced on April 9th that they have approved 20 domestic manufacturers for this task and that they have also ordered shipments of PPE from foreign manufacturers (Pandey, 2020). To further reduce this large deficit of PPE, there have been considerable efforts made by local communities and businesses. For instance, several women-led groups in India have started producing cloth masks and many startup companies have begun 3D printing PPEs (Kadakia, 2020; Pandey, 2020). Moreover, makerspaces in India, such as Maker's Asylum, have also allowed tech enthusiasts to support frontline workers, with 100,000 face shields being produced thus far (Pandey, 2020). However, since the poorer and more remote regions of India do not have access to 3D printing technology, the PPE shortage remains a serious and challenging problem for the Indian government.

Seemingly, despite the large geographical distances between these four countries, there have been some prevalent themes and similarities in the responses to the COVID-19 pandemic. For instance, in many of these countries, the silencing of the concerns of medical professionals appears to be a common theme. This idea can also be seen in countries that neighbour these nations, such as Pakistan, which borders India, and Venezuela, which borders Brazil (Farmer & Wallen, 2020; Watson & Silva). Moreover, another important theme that can be seen is the importance of international cooperation. As previously explained, the implications of an export ban can have deleterious impacts on foreign nations that are reliant on imports. Even the United States, which was one of the many countries that had implemented an export ban, acquires most of their PPE from Asia. Although it is understandable that countries want to protect their own citizens, politicians should carefully consider the humanitarian consequences of their actions as there are many countries that are dependent on imports and may be incapable of manufacturing sufficient amounts of products on their own.

# Chapter 4

## IMPORTANCE OF PREVENTATIVE MEASURES, DISTANCING, AND HARM REDUCTION

As expressed in previous chapters, the unprecedented emergence and rapid spread of COVID-19 in recent times has had severe impacts worldwide and has quickly become the defining global crisis of our time. As of July 18th, 2020, there have been approximately 14.2 million worldwide confirmed cases of COVID-19 and approximately 600,000 deaths as a result of this virus (Johns Hopkins Coronavirus Resource Center, 2020). In Canada, as of July 18th, the government has reported about 110,000 total cases and 8,850 deaths (Government of Canada, 2020a). According to the CDC (Center of Disease Control and Prevention), some symptoms of COVID-19 include fever/chills, cough, shortness of breath, fatigue, congestion, loss of taste/smell, among others (CDC, 2020a). Although the symptoms and implications of the virus itself are not extreme for a healthy person, the coronavirus has a rapid transmissibility rate. Additionally, it presents severe implications for those whose immune systems are compromised; namely, elders and those with pre-existing health and respiratory issues. On March 11th, 2020, WHO declared the coronavirus outbreak a pandemic (Kantis et al., 2020).

Upon the WHO's declaration, several countries around the world have also declared a state of emergency. Promptly, governments and public health systems across nearly every continent implemented lockdowns, travel restrictions, and social distancing measures in attempts to control the spread of the virus, followed suit by the shutdown of various businesses. These measures and shutdowns, albeit having enormous economic and social ramifications, have been crucial in preventing the spread of the virus. Researchers have demonstrated that the virus is primarily spread through being in close contact with an infected person (World Health Organization [WHO], 2020e). Therefore, through ceasing nearly all social interactions as well as encouraging people to practice social distancing, public health systems worldwide have been able to effectively control the rate of spread of the disease.

Currently, as of July 18th, 2020, numerous countries have begun to steadily reopen upon observing the "flattening of the curve" – visual slowing of the rate of spread as a result of preventative public health policies. In Canada, as the number of new cases has begun to decrease over time and the curve continues to flatten, provinces have started to gradually reopen and many local governments have lifted or loosened public health policies such as social distancing, depending on the state of the pandemic in their area (Government of Canada, 2020b). Despite the loosened policies, the national government continues to highlight the importance of practicing safety precautions when going out in public and following preventative measures in order to minimize an individual's risk of infection.

Although local governments have recently started to allow gatherings of a limited number of people, Canadian public health officials still recommend continuing to practice "social distancing", a popular measure that has been implemented by numerous countries ever since the pandemic was declared due to its effectiveness in controlling the rate of spread. Essentially, social distancing entails keeping a safe distance of 2 metres from individuals who do not reside in your household, in both indoor and outdoor areas (Government of Canada, 2020b). This preventative measure helps to limit one's risk of infection as COVID-19 is primarily spread through droplet transmission, which occurs when an individual is in close contact with someone who has respiratory symptoms such as coughing or sneezing. Through being exposed to an infected person's respiratory droplets, this individual is now at risk of becoming infected as well because the mucosae (mouth and nose) and conjunctiva (eyes) are all possible routes of transmission of the coronavirus (WHO, 2020e). As the majority of studies conducted have found that respiratory droplets can travel up to 2 metres from the source (Public Health Ontario, 2020), it is imperative to practice social distancing and maintain a minimum 2 metre gap from others to limit one's exposure to the virus.

The Canadian government also strongly recommends that individuals wear non-medical or cloth masks, especially in settings where it is not possible to maintain a 2 metre distance from others (Government of Canada, 2020b). In addition, many local governments, such as the government of Toronto, have recently enforced policies mandating that people wear face masks in all public enclosed indoor areas, such as public transportation, grocery stores, malls, etc. (DeClerq, 2020). One notable example of the effectiveness of masks happened in Missouri – two hairstylists, after presenting with symptoms of COVID-19, continued to work for several days and saw a total of 139 clients, but none of them became infected. Researchers found that the hairstylists did not infect anyone because they were both wearing masks throughout the period they worked (Young, 2020). Although masks have been proven to be very effective in preventing infected persons from transmitting the virus to others, thus deeming them critical for infected persons to wear, it is unknown how effective face masks are in protecting the healthy wearers from becoming infected. While this information on its own may discourage individuals who do not exhibit symptoms of the virus to wear masks, researchers have recently proven that presymptomatic and asymptomatic transmission can also occur. As these types of transmission occur before or without the onset of symptoms, it is crucial for all people to wear masks in order to protect others – realistically, people could be carrying and spreading the virus without even knowing it.

Presymptomatic transmission occurs when an infected person transmits SARS-CoV-2 to others before he/she develops symptoms, whereas asymptomatic transmission occurs when an infected person transmits SARS-CoV-2 to others despite never developing symptoms. Currently, however, researchers are very unclear about the prevalence and actual plausibility of asymptomatic transmission. The WHO reports that as of April 2nd, 2020, there have been no documented confirmed cases of asymptomatic transmission, although it has been reported during contact tracing in certain countries (WHO, 2020f).

In terms of pre-symptomatic transmission, perhaps the most notable case showcasing the dangers of this type of transmission occurred in Singapore, on January 19th (Shukman, 2020). Upon landing in Singapore, a couple who had flown in from Wuhan, China – which many had believe to be the origin of the coronavirus outbreak

– attended a Sunday service at their local church. They appeared to be healthy and did not demonstrate any symptoms of the virus, however a few days later, the wife became ill, shortly followed by her husband. In the following days, three other people also became infected for seemingly unknown reasons, until it was found that they had attended the church at the same time as the couple; therefore, the couple had spread the virus in spite of having no symptoms at the time. Furthermore, this also emphasizes that there is a critical incubation period of the virus; in this case, the couple became infected approximately 24 to 48 hours prior to the visible display of disease (Shukman, 2020), however, researchers have found that symptoms can take up to 14 days to appear after initial exposure to COVID-19 (Government of Canada, 2020c). Two of the people who became infected were present at the same service as the couple and thus were likely infected via droplet transmission, however, what was perplexing to researchers was the discovery that a third person had also become infected who was not present at the same service. The woman in question had attended a service several hours later, but cameras showed that she had been seated at the same place as the couple during the later service. Thus, researchers hypothesized that the virus had most likely somehow landed on the surface they were seated at (Shukman, 2020). Moreover, this indicates the possibility of another mode of transmission, known as fomite transmission.

Fomite transmission occurs when an infected person releases viral particles onto a surface, effectively contaminating it (Public Health Ontario, 2020). As demonstrated by the Singapore case, it is possible for a healthy individual to become infected by coming into contact with the contaminated surface, likely by touching the surface and subsequently touching their eyes/nose/mouth. In spite of this case, however, there is a lack of real, direct data to prove that infection can occur through contaminated surfaces. There is also a lack of evidence supporting the idea of airborne transmission, which occurs through an infected person's emittance of small particles known as droplet nuclei through coughing, talking, singing, etc. It is believed that droplet nuclei can remain in the air for long periods of time and travel much longer distances than respiratory droplets (WHO, 2020e), however currently, there is no evidence supporting the claim that people can actually contract the virus from droplet nuclei (Public Health Ontario, 2020). In contrast, WHO has reported that some outbreaks occurring in indoor areas may have been caused by a combination of droplet and airborne transmission, thus suggesting that it is valuable to conduct further investigations on the possibilities of airborne transmission particularly in crowded, indoor settings (WHO, 2020h).

As a result of the ambiguities in what modes of transmission are truly viable, in conjunction with the possibility of pre- and asymptomatic transmission, it is absolutely imperative to partake in preventative measures recommended by the government. Researchers are currently uncertain about how effective certain modes of transmission truly are, as they may be dependent upon case by case factors (e.g. setting, immune strength, etc.). Thus, as ongoing research to investigate these ambiguities continues, we must continue to be safe and practice preventative measures, especially now that Canada is gradually reopening. Besides the aforementioned measures of social distancing and using masks, the government of Canada recommends practicing proper personal hygiene via frequently washing your hands for a minimum of 20 seconds with soap and water (or using hand sanitizer in the absence of soap and water), coughing/sneezing into the bend of your arm or a tissue (and promptly disposing the tissue), and avoiding touching your eyes, nose or mouth (Government of Canada, 2020b). In addition to this, the government recommends taking precautionary cleaning measures in order to kill any viral particles that may be present on surfaces. Health Canada recommends using hard surface disinfectants and household cleaners or diluted bleach on commonly touched surfaces such as toilets, phones, electronics, door handles, bedside tables and television remotes (Government of Canada, 2020b).

Aside from these general precautionary guidelines, the Canadian government has also enforced COVID-19-specific harm reduction policies in order to minimize the harm caused by the pandemic towards substance users, particularly opioid users. The opioid epidemic in Canada has been an ongoing public health crisis in which there has been an abundance of opioid overdose deaths and general opioid misuse, often as a result of individuals developing opioid addictions after being prescribed opioids in clinical settings, usually for pain management. The COVID-19 crisis has presented several challenges for individuals affected by the opioid crisis. Lockdowns across the world and lowered income due to layoffs during the pandemic have made it harder for individuals to gain access to drug supplies, thus individuals who are unable to use may experience intense withdrawal symptoms. Furthermore, those who do gain access to supply must use in isolation due to social distancing policies, which increases one's likelihood of overdosing. Additionally, drug users who may become infected by COVID-19 are at heightened risk for developing further health complications or death, as opioid users often have underlying respiratory illnesses (Health Canada, 2020a). As the COVID-19 crisis struck amid the ongoing opioid crisis in Canada, the government has taken crucial steps to limit the damage for individuals who have been caught at the intersection of these two crises (Health Canada, 2020a).

Harm reduction itself is a general term which refers to "strategies and ideas aimed at reducing negative consequences associated with drug use" (Harm Reduction Coalition, n.d.). Furthermore, harm reduction is not intended to shame or denounce those who use substances; rather, it accepts substance use and it instead attempts to minimize the risks of drug use via several strategies (e.g. promoting safe/clean drug usage methods, aiming to improve the well-being and quality of life of drug users rather than focusing on stopping drug use altogether, etc.) (Harm Reduction Coalition, n.d.).

Acknowledging the elevated risks which exist for individuals who use substances during this pandemic, the Canadian government has enforced several temporary harm reduction policies. As many substance user communities are often overcrowded and may lack proper shelter, these communities are particularly susceptible to rapid spread of coronavirus. As a result, Health Canada is allowing provinces and territories to open supervised temporary spaces inside pre-existing consumption sites, thus allowing users to practice social distancing which is often not possible in overcrowded communities (Health Canada, 2020a). Through supervision, these spaces may also diminish an individual's risk of overdose, which often occurs when one engages in isolated drug use. To add to this, Canada has also loosened its standard policies on opioid use in order to align with social distancing policies (e.g. now allowing take-home dosing, allowing pharmacists to extend/renew prescriptions, allowing verbal prescriptions, etc.) (Health Canada, 2020a). In addition, these loosened policies improve users' accessibility to a safe supply of medication, hence decreasing the risks associated with using illegal, toxic supplies. Besides this, several other initiatives have launched, such as the provision of guidelines to healthcare professionals for increasing opioid prescriptions in order to combat symptoms of withdrawal. Resources and support are also being provided to assist drug users who may feel isolated during the pandemic (Health Canada, 2020a).

Conclusively, following preventative public health recommendations have been critical in slowing the spread of the virus, thus it is important to continue to follow these precautionary measures as uncertainties regarding transmission still exist within the scientific field. These preventative measures have been particularly important to follow in the context of protests on social issues such as Black Lives Matter that have been taking place in recent times. As these protests often involve the clustering of many people in concentrated areas, it is essential to practice preventative measures to ensure that you are limiting your risk of infection. Many of these preventative measures involve wearing masks and other personal protective equipment (PPE), however as mentioned in previous chapters, there is a widespread global shortage of PPEs during this pandemic. To address this shortage, there are various global efforts to use 3D printing as an additive manufacturing technique, which will be discussed more in detail in future chapters.

# Chapter 5

## THE HISTORY OF 3D PRINTING TECHNOLOGY

Throughout history, the advancement of technology has not only improved the lives of individuals, but it has also been used to address many global issues. This has especially become apparent with the spread of the COVID-19 pandemic. With this new global issue, many technological advancements have come to light. One type of technology that may appear new, but has a rich history, is 3D printing. Three-dimensional printing brings digital media to life through an additive process where the material is placed in successive layers of the material used. 3D printing has been around for almost 40 years and since its introduction to the world, it has made significant progress in many fields such as medicine (Goldberg, 2018). This is all thanks to Hideo Kodama.

The first prototype of a 3D printer was made by Hideo Kodama in 1981 (Gregurić, 2019b). However, due to problems involving funding, Dr. Kodama did not manage to patent this invention and further innovations were able to be made (Gregurić, 2019b). This included the creation of stereolithography (SLA), a form of 3D printing that was made in 1984 and patented in 1986 by Charles Hull (Gregurić, 2019b). The specific details behind this technology will be discussed in a later chapter, but in essence, stereolithography uses a liquid photopolymer and a computer-generated laser beam to create 3D structures from digital files. At the time of creation, this invention was a huge milestone and advancement for inventors, as it allowed for prototypes to be manufactured easily and cost-effectively. For this reason, in 1988, Charles released SLA-1, a commercial product based upon the process of stereo-lithography (Gregurić, 2019b). Since this technology was newly introduced, there were problems regarding the deformation of the final products.

After the release of SLA-1, another form of 3D printing was introduced in 1988. Selective laser sintering, also known as SLS, was introduced by Carl Decker (Gregurić, 2019b). This process involves the fusion of materials through high-power laser beams (Palermo, 2013a). The generated heat then leads to the fusion of tiny particles of ceramics, glass or plastic to create 3D products (Palermo, 2013a). Interestingly, this technology was not meant to be precise or to create detailed objects, rather created to test this new method in the field of 3D printing. The products made by this technology were mostly chunks of plastic during the early stages of its development. However, in the past several decades, this technology has experienced further development and it is currently still being used in the world of 3D printing.

Following the development of SLS, another form of 3D printing technology was developed by Scott Crump in 1989. This technology is known as fused deposition modeling (FDM) which is commonly recognized as the simplest form of 3D printing (Gregurić, 2019b). In essence, FDM is a process of heating plastic filaments and depositing layers of the material onto a surface to create a 3D model of the digital file. In 1992, Stratasys had issued a patent for the FDM process and this technology had experienced significant levels of development. (Masood, 2014). Due to its simplicity, FDM is now a very well-known 3D printing technology and it has found uses in many different fields, such as engineering, medicine, and academia.

Since the creation of these methods of 3D printing, the possible applications of this technology have exceeded the expectations of many people. This is clearly seen in the year of 1999 as it was a particularly remarkable moment of 3D printing history. Researchers at the Wake Forest Institute for Regenerative Medicine had made a large advancement in the field of bioprinting as they attempted to create a human bladder through 3D printing technology (Siegel, 2019). To further improve the field of bioprinting, an ink-jet printer that would dispense biological ink was later patented by Thomas Boland in 2003. The use of 3D printing in the medical field continues to be extensively researched, especially with the creation of the first bio-printing company, Organovo, in 2007. However, due to the many difficulties involved with bioprinting, such as the large complexities with creating blood vessels, further research is required for the widespread printing of fully functional organs (Moon, 2014).

In addition to the area of organ printing, there have also been many alternatives uses of 3D printing in the medical field, such as using 3D printed models to improve surgery preparation (Nawrat, 2018). With the use of this technology, surgeons are able to view an exact replica of the patient's organ and be able practice before the surgery. This was seen in 2018 as a group of surgeons in Belfast were practicing for a kidney transplant with a 3D printed model (Nawrat, 2018). This may have an enormous potential in the medical field as practice with exact replicas of the patient's organ may allow for safer and more successful surgeries. Additionally, 3D printers have also been used to create surgical instruments. Since the advancement of this technology has allowed for the precise creation of small and accurate instruments, this technology allows for a less invasive approach for operations on smaller areas of the body (Nawrat, 2018). Consequently, this may allow for more precise incisions and it may potentially minimize the amount of scarring on the patient's body. Lastly, the final use of 3D printing technology that will be discussed in this chapter is its use to create custom-made prosthetics. Through the use of 3D printing, the process of creating prosthetics has become significantly faster and less expensive as compared to previously used methods. This technology also allowed patients to model their prosthetics according to the appearance of their limbs, which has been implemented by a system created by Body Labs (Nawrat, 2018). As observed, the impact of 3D printing has been tremendous in the medical field, ranging from allowing custom-made prosthetics at a lower cost to advancing technology in organ printing. As it is clear, 3D printing has played a critical role in the medical field and recent events have shown that the use of this technology will continue to grow.

The spread of COVID-19 has challenged the medical community in a variety of unique ways. Internationally, the shortage of personal protective equipment had demonstrated to be a burden for many medical professionals. With the effects of these shortages becoming more and more severe, many health care providers had resorted to re-using PPE. This presents a huge crisis for health care providers as PPEs are the only form of protection given to those treating COVID-19 patients.

With such vital importance, it is crucial that healthcare facilities are able to maintain an adequate supply of such protection. However, during the past couple months, there have been significant issues surrounding this topic as there were concerns that Canadian imports of PPE would no longer be a viable option.

These concerns first began with the American multinational conglomerate company, 3M, which is largely known for its production of N95 respirators. With the spread of COVID-19, this American company has been responsible for the production of 100 million N95 respirator, one third of which being produced in the US and the rest being produced abroad (McCarten, 2020). However, in April, 3M announced that due to orders from the Trump administration, they have been requested to stop sending their products abroad, more specifically to Canada and Latin America (McCarten, 2020). In response, the Canadian prime minister, Justin Trudeau, announced that it would be a "mistake" for the US to take this step (BBC, 2020). Since Canada does not produce N95 respirators domestically, this could be disastrous for Canadian health facilities and it could sour relations between the two countries. 3M had also spoken out against the request, stating that this would in fact decrease the manufacturing of these masks in the US, since two thirds of the productions take place outside of the country (McCarten, 2020). They also mentioned that this would cause other countries to behave the same way as they may decide to withhold their medical supplies. This was also the topic that Justin Trudeau had spoken out about as he explained that Canada also provides medical equipment for the U.S (BBC, 2020). Therefore, if this request is accepted, there would be a reduction in the back-and-forth trade between the two countries. This situation is now in a calm state as none of the countries acted upon the statements made.

Although PPE imports play a crucial role in maintaining the supply of PPE in health care facilities, domestic production is another important aspect to consider. In March, Justin Trudeau had asked students in colleges, universities, polytechnics and CEGEPS (Collège d'enseignement général et professionnel) for help with the manufacturing of 3D printed PPEs (Boissonneault, 2020). With its highly adaptable manufacturing methods, 3D printing is now a method used all around the world as a means of producing PPE. This can be seen in Canada as many corporations and medical students have started using this technology to create PPE for health care providers. One example of this involves students from McMaster University and the University of Toronto as they had come together to create an organization known as

3D PPE for GTHA (Pearson, 2020). This organization produces face-shields through 3D printing technology and delivers the PPE to medical clinics in Toronto, Hamilton and the Niagara region (Pearson, 2020). This noble act has been widely praised by local communities and many volunteers have flocked to the organization to offer their time and expertise.

Internationally, the use of 3D printing has also been commonly seen in countries all around the world. In February, Wuhan had used 3D printing technology to produce goggles for their medics, manufacturing about 300 units per day (Novak, 2020). In the US, an online platform, known as the NIH 3D Printing Exchange, has partnered with the Food and Drugs Administration (FDA) to gain approval for the use of their PPE designs (Novak, 2020). In the month of June, they had successfully obtained clearance for clinical use and many people began to see the true potential of this technology. As previously mentioned, 3D printing is highly adaptable, allowing manufacturers to produce PPE based on their communities needs while also offering the flexibility to easily make adjustments and improvements (Novak, 2020). This is especially evident with the Prusa face shield, which was developed in the Czech Republic. Following its initial release to the public, the design of this face shield has been updated many times, allowing designers to make the necessary improvements to increase the effectiveness of this product (Novak, 2020). Since adjustments can easily be made with this technology, manufacturers were able to quickly produce the new and improved versions of these face shields. With speed being a key factor during a pandemic, it is evident that 3D printing technology holds enormous potential and it may be the solution to the PPE crisis.

Although 3D printing has been around for about 40 years, it is still considered a new technology. From its humble beginnings of being a method to print media files into crude 3-dimensional objects, such as chunks of plastic, additive manufacturing now a much more refined technology that has the potential to make seemingly science fiction ideas a reality. Beginning with Hideo Kodama's unpatented invention, this journey was quickly followed by Charles Hull with the invention of SLA-1, Carl Decker with the invention of SLS, and Scott Crump with the invention of FDM. Through their work, 3D printing technology has now been able to make monumental contributions in the medical field, including research that could result in the bioprinting of viable organs, the ability to create models of organs that surgeons can use to practice on, the printing of medical equipment, and the customization of prosthetics for individual patients. In addition to these advancements, 3D printing has also been used to support the medical community during the COVID-19 pandemic. With a worldwide shortage of PPEs affecting healthcare professionals across the globe, 3D printing demonstrates significant potential as a possible solution to the crisis.

# **Chapter 6**

## THE 3D PRINTING METHODS OF SLS, SLA AND FDM

After approximately 40 years of technological advancements, the modern additive manufacturing capabilities have surpassed many people's expectations with its wide usage in technological, manufacturing and healthcare industries. To service such a large spectrum of fields and disciplines, a large variety of unique printers have been invented to meet the specific needs of each industry. While some of them specialize in precision and accuracy, others are more cost effective and user friendly. Some may have a smoother surface finish while other printers manufacture objects with better dexterity and durability. With such a large variety in printers, it is important to understand that 3D printing is a broad term that encompasses several manufacturing technologies that build parts layer-by-layer. Each of which varies in the way that it forms plastic and metal parts and can differ in material selection, surface finish, durability, manufacturing speed and cost. In this chapter, the several manufacturing techniques of 3D printing, including Stereolithography (SLA), Selective Laser Sintering (SLS) and Fused Deposition Modeling (FDM), will be discussed and the unique advantages and disadvantages of these techniques will be explored with regards to the manufacturing of PPE during the COVID-19 pandemic. Comparing and contrasting these three types of 3D printing may provide manufacturers, institutions and the public with a solid understanding of what the usage of these three techniques may entail.

Although 3D printing is more widely used for manufacturing prototypes or visualizing models, 3D printing PPE has become much more relevant during this pandemic as it is remarkably cheap and efficient at manufacturing single parts. In this context, single parts may refer to the base structure of a mask, face shield, or a specific component of a hazmat suit. Since the first wave of COVID-19 has already resulted in large scale shortages of PPE, many fear that a second wave could potentially overwhelm the exhausted health care system and put many more frontline workers at risk. However, by rallying local communities and well-established manufacturers to increase the production of PPEs through 3D printing and traditional means, a steady supply of PPE may potentially be achieved in the near future. Although 3D printing technology is normally deployed for smaller volumes of productions, an unprecedented collaboration between 3D printing manufacturers and healthcare institutions may potentially increase the production of 3D printed PPEs and ensure that healthcare facilities are supplied with PPEs that have received proper authorization for safe usage (Ahart, 2019). While the prominence of 3D printing is seen in various aspects of the healthcare industry, it is crucial to understand that the COVID-19 pandemic is an unprecedented situation and that there are many unique considerations that must be made with regards to 3D printing PPE. This includes the costs, quality of raw material, mechanisms and mass production logistics (Ahart, 2019).

To begin, stereolithography (SLA) was the first method of 3D printing to be created (Ahart, 2019). Widely used in the medical industry for human anatomy models, this 3D printing method is known for its precision and accuracy, alongside its smooth finish and durability (Ahart, 2019). This detail-oriented printing procedure allows for better aesthetics as compared to other types of printers and perhaps, would be preferable to the public for fashion forward PPEs like masks and face shields. Some models of 3D printers that use SLA include Vipers, ProJets, and iPros, all of which are sold under the company of 3D Systems, a company known for producing a large range of different 3D printers (Ahart, 2019). To elaborate, the process first begins with instructions from Computer-Aided Designs (CAD) files that may be downloaded from the internet. The printed materials used for SLA are liquid photopolymers, which are a type of plastic that becomes solid after each layer of printing is exposed to an ultraviolet laser (3D Insider, n.d.). This fast process is then followed by a surface blade that evens out the semi-liquid plastic resin and the same process is repeated until the designated object from the CAD file is built completely (3D Insider, n.d.). Afterwards, the completed object is submerged in a chemical bath to remove any excess resin and it is recommended to post-cure the product in an ultraviolet oven for increased durability (3D Insider, n.d.). This fast technology is good for patterns, complex models and production parts due to its low production costs (3D Insider, n.d.). Customized finishes with paint may be an additional cost, but automotive, entertainment and many industries are heavily dependent on this type of 3D printing.

Next, another method of 3D printing known as fused deposition modeling (FDM), is generally used for printing plastic models (Ahart, 2019). Invented by Scott Crump, this particular type of 3D printing rose to prominence through Stratasys Ltd, a very well-known name in the 3D printing industry during the 1980s (Ahart, 2019). Unlike SLA, FDM 3D printing uses production grade thermoplastics to build objects onto a base platform. Depending on the printer and the quality of raw materials, the strength and durability of the 3D printed object will vary. FDM printers often have high precision and accuracy, similar to the characteristics of SLA printers (Ahart, 2019). Consequently, FDM technology is best at producing physical models, proto-types and different types of aids. However, the FDM process is significantly different from SLA as it begins with a specialized software that divides up the 3D CAD files (3D Insider, n.d.). The information is then transferred to the printer, which builds the 3D object layer-by-layer. This involves a high temperature nozzle that deposits the heated thermoplastic mixture onto the base to form the desired product (3D Insider, n.d.). It is noteworthy that other raw materials can be mixed with the ther-moplastic mixture to get a more customized 3D printed object. On the downside, however, a disadvantage to this type of 3D printing is that the 3D objects printed often have rough surface finishes with visible layer lines and they often need to be sanded by hand in order to be usable. Some examples of these FDM printers include the JGAURORA, ALUNAR, and the Original Prusa i3 MK2, but there are many more that exist in the 3D printer market (3D Insider, n.d.). Interestingly, FDM printing is one of the most widely used forms of 3D printing and it has been utilized by large companies, such as BMW and Nestlé (3D Insider, n.d.).

The final 3D printing method that will be discussed in this chapter is selective laser sintering (SLS), which was invented by Dr. Carl Deckard in the 1980's (Ahart, 2019). This type of 3D printing is particularly known for its durability as well as its ability to produce more stable and stronger structures as compared to SLA printing. SLS printing can print with not only thermoplastic materials, but also with white nylon powder, ceramics and glass, which gives this method of 3D printing a versatility like no other (Ahart, 2019). Furthermore, SLS printing does not require structural support during the printing process and can use the whole base platform for a greater surface area for building parts. Generally, SLS is used for manufacturing prototypes and functional testing, but this is also a viable medium for 3D printing PPE (Ahart, 2019). In essence, the process starts with $CO_2$ laser scans on the build platform, which are used to sinter (essentially meaning to solidify) a powdered material (3D Insider, n.d.). With each subsequent scan, the height of the platform is adjusted incrementally, depending on the 3D design, to produce the desired product. During the printing process, the un-sintered powder provides support to the build, but it is eventually removed to extract the printed product. While SLA and SLS are similar in functionality and cost, the difference is that SLA uses a liquid mixture whereas SLS uses powder for 3D printing (3D Insider, n.d.). Some examples of SLA printers include the Nobel 1.0 by XYZprinting, the SUNLU SLA Desktop 3D Printer, and the ProJet 1200 by 3D systems (3D Insider, n.d.).

All three of the techniques that were explored in the previous paragraphs are viable methods of 3D printing that can be used during the pandemic for emergencies. The quality, precision and durability provided by the SLA and SLS printers can accurately mass produce PPE. Depending on the choice of printer, both SLA and SLS printing methods can combinedly use raw materials of plastic as needed, which can contribute to cheaper manufacturing costs. Unfortunately, SLA does require its liquid resins removed and can be burdensome for large volumes of PPE. FDM, on the other hand, produces rough layer lines that may require the PPEs to be individually evaluated and sanded to ensure an acceptable surface finish (3D Insider, n.d.). Since it may be very time consuming to sand down each PPE for large volumes of orders, this can be a limitation to mass manufacturing PPE in such unprecedented circumstances. However, it is noteworthy that FDM and SLS do not require support structures, which is also a great advantage during mass manufacturing.

Fortunately, the designs of face shields and 3D printed masks are not extremely complex, thereby allowing large quantities of these products to be manufactured with relative ease by any of these three methods. However, if complex designs are involved, such as the ones used in hazmat suits, mass manufacturing will be much more challenging as it would result in higher rates of printing errors. According to a scientific article published in the journal Materials, FDM is recommended over SLA for the production of face shields because of the minimal post-printing requirements (Wesemann et al., 2020). By considering the lack of a need for structure support in FDM manufacturing as well as the fact that face shields have a relatively simple design, the authors concluded that FDM would be a more appropriate approach for this specific type of PPE (Wesemann et al., 2020). However, the recommendations for the methods of 3D printing will vary with different PPEs as there would be significant differences in the complexity and specific requirements involved.

While 3D printed PPE, especially masks and shields, may be able to tackle the shortage in different developed and developing countries battling COVID-19, their level of safety and protection is being improved everyday as new designs and companies come forth to collaborate. To give numbers in this context, 500,000 3D printed face shields and over 348,000 masks were deployed for healthcare workers and vulnerable groups (U.S. Food and Drug Administration [FDA], 2020a). Moreover, comparing and contrasting these three types of 3D printing provides a fair estimate of their compatibility for making PPE but it is extremely important to emphasize the need for approval by government regulated organizations or healthcare institutions before regular use. In the US, the FDA has attempted to regulate this process by providing regulations and checklists to many companies that have come forward to help produce PPE (FDA, 2020a). To support this initiative, FDA is currently working with National Institute of Health (NIH) and Veteran Affairs (VA) to provide assistance for manufacturing PPE through 3D printing, which speaks to the credibility and capabilities of 3D printing by companies and individuals (FDA, 2020a).

In summary, SLS, SLA and FDM all have their own unique advantages and disadvantages with regards to mass manufacturing PPE. Since these attributes are often situational, it is important for the 3D printing community to choose the appropriate approach for the specific type of PPE that they are manufacturing. In order to ensure that volunteers and manufacturing companies are provided with sufficient information to make this decision, further research exploring the various 3D printing techniques for each type of PPE needs to be conducted so that scientifically supported recommendations can be made available to the public. However, it should be noted that there are several countries that lack 3D printing capabilities, let alone the option between SLA, FDM, and SLS. With many of these countries suffering from widespread PPE shortages, countries in the developed world may want to recognize their privilege and use this technology for the betterment of the world.

# Chapter 7

## POLYMER JET FABRICATION

In the early 2000s, the prominence of 3D printing skyrocketed in the medical industry (Goldberg, 2020). Starting with the components for internal organs and eventually creating full functioning kidneys, 3D printing has grown and developed exponentially in the healthcare industry as a result of its efficiency and cost effectiveness. The Wake Forest Institute 3D printed the first human bladder scaffold surrounding the synthetic body (Goldberg, 2020). Additionally, a company in San Francisco called Bespoke Innovations created personalized 3D printed legs for amputees to match every individual's body symmetry (Goldberg, 2020). Although the famous RepRap Project by Dr. Adrian Bower assembled a printer with mostly 3D printed parts, since then, many other businesses and industries have followed this phenomenon (Goldberg, 2020). A case in point being that many countries' aviation and automotive industries use 3D printed industrial parts for mass manufacturing and accuracy. Evidently, the usage of 3D printing is very versatile and has become widespread across various industries in recent times, particularly the medical industry. Therefore, when the COVID-19 pandemic led to a shortage of Personal Protective Equipment (PPE), which includes products such as facemasks, face shields, gloves and suits, many companies creatively turned to 3D printing as a temporary solution. Globally, over 1700 3D printing specialists have offered to help make protective equipment for hospitals during this pandemic (Gregurić, 2019a). While SLS and FDM may be more commonly used, polymer jet fabrication is another method of 3D printing that has recently become popular amongst many industries.

Polymer Jet Fabrication technology, also known as PolyJet technology, uses millions of photopolymer liquid droplets which it 'jets' onto a build platform, steadily building a structure, followed

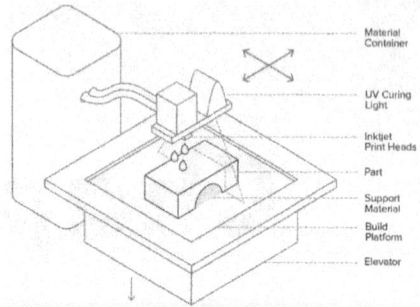

Material Container

UV Curing Light

Inkjet Print Heads

Part

Support Material

Build Platform

Elevator

by a ray of UV light which stabilizes the structure printed (Gregurić, 2019a). The three stages of polymer jet fabrication are known as: pre-processing, production and support removal (Proto3000, 2020). The pre-processing stage involves a software known as 3D Computer Aided Design (CAD) which decides the photopolymer arrangement, the duration of UV light exposure, and the aesthetic properties of the product like colour and texture (Proto3000, 2020). A 3D CAD file is generally used for the visualization of 3D models or designs, created by the CAD software for 3D printing purposes. The next step is production, which entails the printing of the photopolymers in thin layers and subsequent curing with UV light (Proto3000, 2020). The printer itself is made up of several parts, including a materials container, a build platform and a carriage with spaces for UV light and printing jets. Photopolymers are usually heated to a temperature ranging from 30 to 60°C and poured into the materials container for easy spraying of the photopolymer droplets (Proto3000, 2020). The viscosity, concentration and microstructures of the photopolymer are important for smooth printing (Gregurić, 2019a). The printing carriage sprays photopolymers across the X-axis of the build platform in an arrangement which was predetermined by the CAD file, and the UV light cures the structure to solidify it. The act of spraying the 3D printed lines across the x-axis is also known as Line-Wise deposition. Support removal for the newly 3D printed structure either by hand, with water, or with solution.

In the year 2000, a company called Object Geometries developed the first PolyJet printer with their name on various patents (Gregurić, 2019a). While the aforementioned mechanism of photopolymers and UV light is standardized across all printers which use this method of 3D printing, different companies name and brand their printers differently in order to claim their rights on patents. For example, in 2011, when the company Stratasys took over Object Geometries, they changed the name of this 3D printer product line to MultiJet, where it was previously known as PolyJet for Object Geometries, even though the differences between the renamed printer and original printer are very minimal and insignificant; both are essentially the same technology (Gregurić, 2019a; Proto3000, 2020). To delve deeper, the only minor technical difference between PolyJet and MultiJet is the support material which is left over after 3D printing different structures. While PolyJet uses dissolvable support material (such as glycerin, propylene, and polyethylene), MultiJet uses paraffin wax which requires an oven to be melted after 3D printing (Gregurić, 2019a; Proto3000, 2020). Fortunately, the PolyJet's leftover materials can be removed with water or by hand and be dissolved into a chemical solution for reuse.

The Polymer Jet fabrication method of 3D printing demonstrates remarkably fast and accurate results, which attests to its capability of producing intricate pieces of technology such as printers, complex models, robots, plastic organs, dental moulds, and medical equipment. Some of the special features of polymer jet fabrication include precise strokes, smooth prints, ability to print different shapes, and detailed presentation as a result of its ability to mix customized concentrations of photopolymers (Proto3000, 2020). Furthermore, the PolyJet technology is able to print 3D structures and microstructures with a wide selection of colours, ranging from dull, pastel colours to bright, vibrant shades (Proto3000, 2020). With over 1000 material properties (color and texture) to choose from, printing models of detailed textures and patterns are not a strenuous process for this machine (Proto3000, 2020). In contrast, the biggest disadvantage of this machine is the fact that due to its complex parts and the large range of materials used for 3D printing, the price is relatively high. Despite the vast capabilities and advantages of this technique of 3D printing, there are still some limitations and concerns. As the PolyJet/MultiJet printers are one of the newest forms of 3D printing with small scale production capability, many question the durability of its printed parts (Gregurić, 2019a). Many 3D printing methods are known to produce fragile products, like Stereolithography (SLA), which raises speculations about the effectiveness of Polymer Jet fabrication as well.

PolyJet 3D printing appeals to a variety of professions and industries. As a result of its ability to create intricate and detailed replicas of human parts, recently polymer jet fabrication has been used frequently by health professionals in the medical industry. Medical education across Canada has been enhanced by the usage of life-like models such as complex tissues, muscle fibres and blood vessels. Furthermore, architects and interior designers can also take advantage of PolyJet printing by designing 3D printable models of buildings and interiors with a great amount of detail, allowing clear communication with clients. Since 3D printing was invented, many tech industries have utilized this technology for making several products such as machine parts, robots and complex models. Now, with the relatively recent invention of PolyJet technology, they can be even more accurate with functional prototypes and efficiency. Whether it is the aerospace, defense or automotive industry, various companies like HP, Proto Labs and Stratasys are able to generate billions of dollars in revenue using 3D printing technology (Alspach, 2019). Considering its colossal expansion into a wide range of industries including the medical industry, 3D printing has recently been used as a means by which companies can help tackle the crisis of medical equipment shortages efficiently. For instance, in Canada, a company named INKsmith scaled up its employment in order to increase production of face shields and masks (Shieber, 2020). Smaller companies have also contributed to the PPE manufacturing effort, such as Markforged and Brooklyn's Voodoo Manufacturing in the U.S. A New York based non-profit organization called COVID Maker Response has delivered over 19 000 face shields through 3D printing to about 50 healthcare facilities (Statt, 2020).

Upon the official announcement of COVID-19 as a pandemic, governments, hospital institutions and everyday citizens began to panic. At the beginning of the pandemic, several individuals stockpiled PPE in fright, which consequently led to the shortages of PPE in hospitals and other healthcare institutions. However, fortunately, many private and international companies and corporations have efficiently used their resources to try to meet the seemingly never-ending demands. Social media and personal initiatives have played a huge role in overcoming the shortage of PPE. Statistics show that 20% of conversations on various social media platforms consisted of topics related to COVID-19 and the shortages of PPE (Vordos et al., 2020). Seeing people's widespread concern across the internet, tech companies, university institutions, pharmaceutical companies and COVID-19 response organizations were encouraged to use 3D printing as a creative solution. The United States of America possesses over 444 000 3D printers, followed by the United Kingdom and Germany (Vordos et al., 2020). Vordos and colleagues (2020) have discussed the potential of using 3D printers to their full capacity in a given country in order to combat the PPE crisis. For example, with about 500 3D printers, Greece can supply over 6000 face shields in just a few days (Vordos et al., 2020). If countries like the US use their 3D printers to full capacity, perhaps PPE could be replenished more rapidly. Furthermore, using technology such as Polymer Jet fabrication and MultiJet technology can make more complex and intricate equipment than other 3D printing techniques, like creating detailed and customized shields, respirators, visors, nebulizers and ventilators (Vordos et al., 2020). The increase in efficiency would peak if PolyJet printers were used instead of stereolithography because it is efficient and versatile. Indeed, the Food and Drug Administration (FDA) in the U.S. has allowed 3D printed equipment to be used in medical facilities given that all criteria and validation procedures are followed, thus allowing 3D printing to be used as an efficient tool to help reduce PPE shortages (U.S. Food and Drug Administration [FDA], 2020d).

Conversely, controversies regarding 3D printed equipment arose in the medical community soon after the introductions of 3D printed masks and face shields. While effective and efficient, Polymer Jet fabrication may not be able to provide the necessary protection as clinically certified N95 respirators or certified face masks with specially engineered electrostatic barriers to catch the smallest of particles. The filtration system and materials used in PolyJet printing may not be able to prevent the transmission of harmful microscopic bacteria or viruses. The Massachusetts Institute of Technology advises manufacturers to not mass produce PPE with 3D printing within the university, but instead only use 3D printers for making prototypes (Gallagher, 2020). Despite the immense benefits that 3D printing can provide in times of shortage, many health-related efficacy issues are yet to be addressed. 3D printed materials may be combustible and thus hazardous when in contact with sterile chemicals and heat, which are both often present in various healthcare facilities (Gallagher, 2020). A possible approach to solve this dilemma can be attempting to incorporate the raw materials used in FDA-certified masks and PPE companies. Injection molding can be used to mass manufacture plastic products, which should be utilized to its full potential for making face shields, however PolyJet should be utilized for manufacturing more sophisticated, intricate medical equipment (Gallagher, 2020). Tech giants like HP have partnered with various companies and institutions, namely Chicago's Fast Radius and The Czech Institute of Informatics, to mass manufacture face masks, respirators, and a plethora of other medical parts through 3D printing and distributed them in hospitals and communities with shortages for Personal Protective Equipment (PPE) (Petch, 2020). These companies are ensuring the safe usage and standards of the PPE by abiding by FDA regulations and guidelines for emergency PPE manufacturing (FDA, 2020d). Although the filter media is a point of concern in 3D printed PPE, recently PolyJet printing has been utilizing many materials which are identical to those used in the regular manufacturing of PPE. Furthermore, ideas for future enhancements for 3D printers in the medical field are well on their way, thus 3D printing can potentially progress towards manufacturing virtually impermeable, certified medical-grade PPE in the future. With its fleet of MutiJet, which again, uses nearly identical technology as PolyJet printers, it was possible to mass manufacture PPE, with the help of healthcare institutions and companies.

In the final analysis, considering its pros and cons of PolyJet, it is evident that 3D printing has been significantly favoured to manufacture PPE by the majority of the governments and institutions, with the approval of the FDA and governing authorities like Health Canada. Ishack and Lipner (2020) have discussed the possible changes and reinforcements that can be made in 3D printed respirators to meet the standards of medical-grade N95 respirators. To be compatible with 3D printing, a mix of polypropylene (PP) and styrene-(ethylene-butylene)-styrene (SEBS) can be used as this material effectively replicates the protective barrier found in N95 respirators (Ishack & Lipner, 2020). As a lot of these suggested improvements involve working with such complex designs and materials, amongst other printing methods, PolyJet or MultiJet printers would be ideal in creating such intricate designs and complex textures (involving two or more raw materials). PolyJet printers can also easily utilize the same raw materials as regular face shields, such as polycarbonate, polyester, and polyvinyl chloride in order to meet the increased demands of PPE during this pandemic (Ishack & Lipner, 2020). Another equipment for which PolyJet and MultiJet printers can be used are ventilator valves. Instead of reusing expensive ventilators for all admitted patients, which can be hazardous if improper sterilization techniques are employed, 3D printing can create disposable ventilator valves which can be much safer and cheaper (Ishack & Lipner, 2020). Moreover, PolyJet printers can also be mobilized to mass produce medications and vaccines, because conventional medicine-printing technology mirrors the mechanism of 'jetting' with a nozzle or spray to make pills (Ishack & Lipner, 2020). More research and development should be dedicated towards 3D printing, specifically PolyJet printing, in the medical field in case of future epidemics or outbreaks.

The rapid depletion of PPE during this unprecedented pandemic has shown us the power of 3D printing technology as a means of mass manufacturing PPE. Polymer Jet Fabrication, particularly, embodies the efficiency, durability and versatility to be used in the manufacturing of PPE from masks to ventilators. The wide usage and accessibility of PolyJet 3D printing in this crisis has led the maker community to lend a helping hand to hospital facilities and health institutions in need. Many people from home have also utilized their personal PolyJet 3D printers, especially in the US, to help supply hospitals with face shields and masks, creating a chain of community collaboration (Ishack & Lipner, 2020). With advice and expertise from many government officials and doctors, whether it is regular PPE or PolyJet 3D printed PPE, it is recommended to utilize PPE to cover your mouth and nose and practice other preventative measures against COVID-19. Mass producing PolyJet 3D printed PPE will undoubtedly lend a helping hand to companies struggling to meet the demands of the public.

# **Chapter 8**

## INJECTION MOLDING

In 1872, the manufacturing process known as injection molding was first developed by John Wesley Hyatt (J. S. Hyatt & J. W. Hyatt, 1872). Interestingly, the events leading up to this innovation began with a rising concern of the rapidly declining population of elephants (Seeger, 2011). As ivory was highly sought-after material that was used in the production of various products, the growing middle class had only increased the demand for this scarce commodity (Seeger, 2011). This potential ivory shortage had proved to be a major concern for Phelan and Collander, a billiard ball manufacturing company, as billiard balls were manufactured from ivory during the 19th century. To tackle this issue, the company offered a $10,000 prize for a substitute for ivory (White, 1999). This led Hyatt to investigate and develop a nitrocellulose-camphor compound known as Celluloid (White, 1999). This material is regarded as the first man-made plastic and its discovery led Hyatt to patent many new inventions involving the manufacturing and processing of plastic products. One such invention was the world's first injection molding machine, which molded plastic products from celluloid (J. S. Hyatt & J. W. Hyatt, 1872; White, 1999). This innovation revolutionized the plastic manufacturing industry and through further improvements made by James Watson Hendry, plastic products could be manufactured with greater speed and higher quality (Arrowsmith, 2014).

Currently, injection molding is the most common process of manufacturing plastic components and it is heavily employed by the automotive, appliance, technology, and recreation and toy industries, among many others. In essence, injection molding is a cyclic process that involves the injection of melted plastic into a mold to produce a plastic product with the desired shape (Benitez-Rangel et al., 2007; Bennett, 2018; Santa Clara University Engineering Design Center, n.d.). This cycle can be divided into the four stages: clamping, injection, cooling, and ejection and the machine responsible for facilitating this process consists of the clamping unit, the injection unit, and the mold (CustomPartNet, n.d.; Polyplastics, n.d). Beginning with the first stage of clamping, the clamping unit is used to securely close the two halves of the mold (CustomPartNet, n.d.). Next, plastic pellets are fed into the injection unit where the pellets melted into a molten state by the heating bands (Benitez-Rangel et al., 2007). During this time, a screw inside of the injection unit is rotated to exert a force towards the mold where the molten plastic would accumulate (CustomPartNet, n.d.; Polyplastics, n.d). Once the molten plastic has reached sufficient levels, the plastic is then injected into the mold cavity where the cooling stage may begin (Rezai et al., 2012). This cooling process allows the plastic to solidify into the desired shape and after a sufficient amount of time, the mold is then reopened to allow for ejection (Rezai et al., 2012). Once the final plastic product is ejected out of the mold, the clamping unit can then reclose the two halves of the mold to repeat this injection molding process (Benitez-Rangel et al., 2007; Rezai et al., 2012).

Through the years, injection molding has been widely praised for its efficiency and it has maintained its status as being one of the most important manufacturing processes capable of mass production (Chen & Turng; Bennett, 2018). However, in the past few decades, many manufacturers have been turning their attention to the new and innovative technology of 3D printing. In the United States alone, the amount spent on 3D printing has gone from approximately $800 million in 2005 to $4.2 billion in 2015 (Franchetti & Kress, 2016). This significant increase can largely be attributed to improvements in affordability in recent decades (Franchetti & Kress, 2016). With these decreased costs, 3D printing has grown to be an increasingly enticing approach for manufacturing. Unlike injection molding, 3D printing is highly cost-effective for small scale production and it has relatively low fixed costs (Berman, 2012). With injection molding, the costs associated with designing, engineering, and manufacturing the mold can be very expensive (Redwood, n.d.; Reeves

& Merlus, 2017). These costs can range from thousands to hundreds of thousands of dollars and once the molds are produced, they are incredibly difficult to modify (Pomager, 2015). Consequently, manufacturers using injection molding are often required to produce large quantities of products as it would be financially unfeasible to use this technology for small scale production (Berman, 2012; Redwood, n.d.). However, there is also a financial risk associated with large scale production as an insufficient demand for the product could result in low inventory turnover and high storage costs (Berman, 2012). Since 3D printing does not require the large initial investment of an expensive mold, there is a significantly lower setup cost associated with 3D printing (Berman, 2012; Franchetti & Kress, 2016; Redwood, n.d.). This enables 3D printing to be financially viable at low scale production and it also makes it feasible for products to be manufactured at an as-needed basis, thereby mitigating the risk of low inventory turnover (Berman, 2012).

Although it may appear that 3D printing and injection molding are in competition against each other, these two manufacturing processes may also be used alongside one another to optimize production (Jahan & El-Mounayri, 2016; Redwood, n.d.; Yang et al., 2017). As previously mentioned, injection molding is often used to manufacture large quantities of products. Consequently, the molds are frequently subject to large amounts of stress, which can partly be attributed to the repeated action of opening and closing the mold as well as the exposure to the pressures and temperatures of the molten plastic (Brezinová & Guzanová, 2009; Redwood, n.d). For this reason, injection molds are often manufactured from metals, such as aluminum and steel, as these materials provide the mold with wear resistance (Redwood, n.d). However, when producing small quantities of goods, the importance of wear resistance rapidly decreases as the mold would be exposed to a significantly lower amount of stress (Redwood, n.d.). Thus, manufacturers would be able to cut production costs by choosing to use a weaker, but significantly cheaper material for small scale production. An increasingly popular example of this kind of mold is 3D printed molds (McGuigan, 2020; Styles, 2018).

Despite the fact that 3D printed molds are only capable of producing approximately 100 parts before they are rendered unusable, these 3D printed molds can be manufactured in roughly a day while traditional metal molds require several weeks (Hanson, 2019). This substantially shorter time period paired with its significantly lower setup costs makes 3D printed molds a very appealing alternative. In addition,

3D printed molds present another major incentive as the mold design could be modified at almost no extra cost (The Economist, 2011). As previously mentioned, this contrasts with the traditional metal molds, which are highly difficult and expensive to modify once they are produced (Chen, 2020). This advantage eliminates the financial risk associated with investing in an expensive metal mold and it presents manufacturers with a newfound confidence to produce injection molds without fearing the possibilities of future modifications (Redwood, n.d). Furthermore, 3D printed molds can be particularly useful for manufacturing functional prototypes (Pomager, 2015). Although prototypes can be produced directly through 3D printing, the materials intended for the manufacturing of the final product are commonly incompatible with 3D printing (Pomager, 2015). This presents an issue for product developers as the prototypes produced from 3D printed material often demonstrate considerable differences from the final product, thereby causing it to be unsuitable for accurate functional testing (Pomager, 2015). However, this issue could be avoided by using 3D printed injection molds (Pomager, 2015). Since injection molding allows prototypes to be produced from the intended material, manufacturers can produce functional prototypes in a short period of time by 3D printing the injection molds (Pomager, 2015). This can be particularly useful when time is of the essence as it would allow products to be tested and potentially approved at an earlier time. Evidently, the advantageous qualities of 3D printing and injection molding can be further enhanced by using these technologies to complement each other.

As with all manufacturing processes, 3D printing injection molds have their own critiques and drawbacks. One common criticism of 3D printing is that the surface finish quality of 3D parts is poor (Styles, 2018). This can present a large concern for 3D printed molds as the poor surface finish would be able to transfer onto the plastic product. However, recently, there have been major improvements regarding the surface finish quality of 3D printed parts and currently, there are certain technologies, such as Polymer Jet Fabrication and Stereolithography, that have been reported to be capable of producing parts with an excellent surface finish (Redwood, n.d; Styles, 2018). Additionally, another major criticism of 3D printed molds is the poor thermal conductivity of plastic (Chen, 2020). Since plastic is an insulator, 3D printed molds have a longer heating and cooling phase as compared to the traditional metal molds (Chen, 2020). Consequently, this would decrease the efficiency and cost-effectiveness of injection molding as the increase in cycle time would result in a decrease in the number of products that can be produced within a given time period (Chen, 2020; Styles, 2018). However, to address this issue, manufacturers can incorporate thermal conductive additives, such as boron nitride and iron particles, into the mold material (Chen, 2020). This would improve the thermal conductivity of the 3D printed mold, thereby decreasing the cycle time as well as addressing the negative implications that were previously mentioned.

With regards to the ongoing COVID-19 pandemic, many companies and volunteers have seen the potential applications of 3D printing and injection molding technologies. As mentioned in the previous chapters, the increased demand for PPE has resulted in widespread shortages (WHO, 2020c). To meet this demand, multi-billion dollar corporations and philanthropic volunteers have attempted to support frontline workers by 3D printing PPE as well as ventilator parts. Cisco, for instance, had collaborated with the Yale Center for Engineering Innovation and Design (CEID) to support the Yale School of Nursing with 3D printed PPE (Yale School of Nursing [YSN], 2020). Through the hard and charitable work of over 150 volunteers, this collaboration had yielded approximately 10,000 face shields in their best week (YSN, 2020). Seemingly, 3D printing has demonstrated that it can have an enormous impact in emergency situations, and it has allowed for a large community effort to help tackle the widespread PPE shortages. However, it is important to note that this has not been the only use of 3D printing during the COVID-19 pandemic as there have been many companies that have started using 3D printed injection molds to manufacture PPEs.

As previously mentioned, these plastic molds can be produced in a substantially lower amount of time than the traditional metal molds. This allows manufacturers to utilize injection molding technology relatively early on, thereby allowing PPEs to be manufactured quickly as well as enabling the fast production of functional prototypes. The latter can be especially important during a pandemic setting because the faster a functional prototype can be produced, the faster it can undergo testing and be approved for medical use. Although it was prior to the pandemic, this was seen with OBMedical, a company that manufactures medical devices. The 3D printed injection mold for one of their products had allowed the company to quickly obtain a functional prototype to perform safety tests on (Pomager, 2015). This had allowed the company to finish testing its prototype and file for FDA clearance in a much shorter period of time than initially anticipated (Pomager, 2020).

With COVID-19 cases continuing to rise throughout the world, the sooner effective machines and equipment can be approved for use, the more lives that can possibly be saved.

Although the current efforts to 3D print PPE have been particularly successful with regards to being a quick response to the shortages, 3D printing would not be an effective long-term solution (Gitlin, 2020). Despite being a highly cost-effective technology for low volume production, the same cannot be said about large scale production. In contrast to traditional mass manufacturing techniques, such as injection molding, large scale production involving 3D printing entails a higher cost per part and requires more time to manufacture each product (Berman, 2012; Styles, 2018; Thompson, 2020). However, as previously mentioned, metal injection molds require several weeks to manufacture, which is an incredibly long period of time to wait for the frontline workers. For this reason, many manufacturers, such as General Motors, have been 3D printing PPEs as a temporary measure until the injection molds are ready for mass production (Gitlin, 2020). Thus, 3D printing should not be viewed as a replacement for injection molding processes, but rather a complementary tool to allow for a much more effective response.

Evidently, 3D printing and injection molding can have an enormous impact during a pandemic setting. In situations where there is a high sense of urgency, 3D printing is capable of rapidly responding to the crisis. Whether this is done through 3D printing the equipment directly or through the production of 3D printed injection molds, the fast response of 3D printing can help alleviate the crisis and fill in the gaps in the supply chains. In the long run, however, injection molding should be prioritized instead as it is a more effective process for large scale production. Seemingly, instead of treating 3D printing and injection molding as separate solutions to the crisis, a more effective approach would be to use the two technologies in combination so that they can complement each other's strengths. This concerted effort can provide a highly efficient and cost-effective solution to the widespread PPE shortages that have plagued the world.

# Chapter 9

## STAMPING

Stamping, also commonly referred to as pressing, is a manufacturing process which uses flat metal sheets and transforms them into distinct shapes and products. (Mills, 2015; Engineering Specialities, Inc. [ESI], n.d.). More specifically, this process involves flat metal sheets being fed into a machine called a stamping press, in which a 'tool and die' surface molds the metal into a desired shape (Mills, 2015). The 'tool and die' surface refers to a specialized precision tool known as a stamping die. Various different types of stamping dies exist, and different dies utilize different operations in order to mold and construct the metal product. Stamping dies are made of a particular type of hardenable steel known as tool steel, hence the name 'tool and die' (Hedrick, 2018). Typically, stamping is used as a metalworking process (works on metal sheets), however stamping can also sometimes be used to manufacture products made of other materials such as paper, leather and rubber (Mills, 2015). Stamping presses are also mainly powered in three different ways – mechanical, which uses a motor connected to a mechanical flywheel (spinning of the wheel produces energy to power the press), hydraulic, in which the stamping press is powered via pressurized hydraulic fluid, and mechanical servo, in which the stamping press is powered via high capacity motors (Mills, 2015). As it is the least expensive of the three methods, stamping presses are most commonly powered via a mechanical flywheel (Mills, 2015).

Historically, stamping has had a rather intriguing background. Upon the discovery of different metals, mankind had been attempting to figure out how to shape and mold metal for centuries. It is believed that the first evidence of the initial development of the stamping technique was coins. The ancient Lydians in seventh century BC were the first people to implement the basic methods of stamping in order to create designs on coins – this essentially entailed carving an image into a stamp and hammering it onto the coin (Thomas Engineering Company, 2015). The hammering method became the standardized process of creating coins until 1550, when a German silversmith named Marx Schwab further advanced the stamping technique through developing a process involving a screw press (Thomas Engineering Company, 2015). Fundamentally, the screw press is a manually powered machine which could sometimes take up to twelve men turning a wheel in order to generate the force needed to stamp the coins. In spite of the heavy manpower required, Schwab's creation was more precise and consistently accurate in the placement of the stamp than the previous hammering procedure (Thomas Engineering Company, 2015).

Later on, with the onset of the industrial revolution, all manufacturing processes became more automated and thus steam power was used rather than manual power to lift heavy weights which were used to stamp designs onto coins. Coin stamping techniques continued to advance as a result of technological advances, however stamping was not actually applied to constructing industrial metal parts until 1890, when Germany began using metal stamping to create bicycle parts (Thomas Engineering Company, 2015). This led to the recognition of metal stamping as a common industrial manufacturing process, as people began to observe that it was an efficient and relatively inexpensive process. Today, metal stamping is a standardized industrial process that is used to manufacture a wide variety of products, ranging from airplane parts to medical equipment.

As mentioned previously, stamping transforms metal sheets via a stamping press. Essentially, a stamping press is a machine with two halves – the lower half is a surface on which the metal sheet is placed, and the upper half uses a stamping die to strike the metal and shape it (Bozard, n.d.). Several different kinds of stamping dies exist, all of which perform different operations. Notably, punching, blanking, embossing, and coining are a few examples of common operations performed by stamping dies (Mills, 2015). Punching and blanking are cutting operations which are essentially inverse versions of each other – both involve cutting a circle in the metal sheet, but punching uses the outer portion of the metal sheet as the product (leaving the circle as scrap), whereas blanking uses the hole as the product (leaving the outer metal sheet as scrap) (Mills, 2015). Embossing and coining, on the other hand, are operations which are used to stamp designs into the metal sheet. In embossing, a design is pressed into the metal sheet via a stamping die which contains the desired design. On the other hand, in coining, the metal sheet is placed between a stamping die and the press, allowing the tip of the press to penetrate and create bends in the metal – as its name suggests, coining is typically used to create coins (Mills, 2015). Stamping presses are usually programmed to perform a specific operation (e.g. punching, coining, etc.) using computer-aided design (CAD) software. Once the software has been developed, craftsmen called diemakers translate it into a physical stamping die (Mills, 2015).

There are also various different ways in which stamping presses are organized in factories, known as stamping techniques. Perhaps the most common stamping technique is progressive die stamping, which is a sequential process (ESI, n.d.). Stamping presses are placed in a specific order and each press performs a definitive function as the metal continuously moves horizontally along the press. Each press progressively transforms the metal in a different way, successively contributing to the final product (ESI, n.d.; Mills, 2015). Progressive die stamping enables easy repeatability and fast production; hence it is ideally suited for creating metal parts with complex geometry (Mills, 2015). Similarly, transfer die stamping is a technique which uses a sequential process analogous to progressive die stamping, with the key difference in this technique being that each stamping press is placed at a distance from the others rather than one after the other. Upon one stamping press completing its operation on the metal sheet, a conveyor belt is used to transport the metal to the next press (Mills, 2015). As this process is relatively slow compared to progressive die stamping, transfer die stamping is typically used for the production of larger parts (Mills, 2015).

Stamping is used to manufacture a variety of mainly metal products, ranging from small, simplistic objects, such as metal clips and washers, to large, complex machinery, such as engine bases and parts of home appliances (Mills, 2015). As it has relatively lower production costs, lower labour costs and easier automation compared to other common manufacturing processes, stamping is used to construct products across a vast range of industries. Markedly, some of these industries include the aerospace industry, telecommunications services, military and defense, microelectronics, and most significantly for our context, medical equipment manufacturers (Mills, 2015). Since metals are generally the material used for stamping, rather than personal protective equipment (PPE), stamping is usually used to manufacture products such as surgical instruments, temperature probes, device pumps, and implantable devices (Pacific Metal Stampings, n.d.). Although stamping occasionally works on paper and rubber as well, it is quite uncommon for stamping manufacturers to use a material other than metal. Thus, it is quite rare for personal protective equipment (PPE) to be generated via stamping presses, but it is still possible.

Conversely, as discussed in previous chapters, 3D printing has been used in abundance to produce PPE for COVID-19 in recent times, as a result of the widespread PPE shortages in various countries globally. According to a Global News article from April, volunteers across Canada have been using 3D printers in their possession to produce PPE and other essential equipment in order to withstand the shortages and support frontline workers during the pandemic (Thompson, 2020). There are also a variety of other 3D printing initiatives around the world, namely the US. Evidently, 3D printing has been very effective in consistently combatting shortages and protecting people during this pandemic.

In general, there has been a great deal of ongoing debate surrounding the potential of 3D printing to replace pre-existing standardized manufacturing techniques, such as stamping. In terms of accuracy, 3D printing is much more automated and requires little to no human intervention aside from creating the initial 3D-printable design. Contrarily, stamping often requires multiple operators along the assembly line, as well as supervisors to perform quality checks during the manufacturing process (Bozard, n.d.). As a result, it is arguable that 3D printing ensures more accuracy in manufacturing products as it is subject to less human error. In addition, 3D printers are not as bulky as stamping presses and occupy less space than stamping plants. Therefore, more products could be manufactured within the same amount of space, thereby maximizing output (Bozard, n.d.). From an environmental perspective, 3D printers are also comparatively much less wasteful. Many metal stamping operations involve starting off with a sheet of metal and cutting it to form the desired final product, generating wasted scrap material, while 3D printers fold layers of material together so that no material is wasted.

Furthermore, when comparing cost, as 3D printers are automated and comparatively take up very little space, products can easily be manufactured locally using 3D printers, hence eliminating the cost of shipping and other human-mediated logistic activities. Although the initial setup cost of 3D printers can be quite high due to the high unit cost of 3D printers, costs are cut in other areas (e.g. lower labour costs, less wastage of material, lower or no shipping cost, etc.), so the overall cost is still lower (Rathi, 2018). In addition, 3D printers are much more easily customizable and adaptable than stamping presses. To create a new design using stamping, new dies would have to be created, which creates additional labour and manufacturing costs. On the other hand, in 3D printing, customization is very simple as new designs can be created digitally, which does not generate any additional costs. There is also no added cost for creating products with more complicated designs – whether printing a complex design or simplistic design, if both products are of the same size, the cost will be nearly the same (Rathi, 2018). Thus, there is a large versatility of possible products that can be made using a 3D printer without any additional costs.

In spite of these advantages, 3D printers still have several limitations in comparison to stamping presses. Namely, while 3D printers can produce an extensive variety of products, they take longer to manufacture small, simple parts, such as washers – stamping is much more efficient in terms of manufacturing plain parts (Bozard, n.d.). As a result, 3D printers are more suitable for manufacturing more intricate products, whereas stamping presses are better suited towards creating uncomplicated, conventional parts. Besides this, many argue that 3D printing, albeit its emergence as an innovative technology, still has its limitations in terms of product quality because it is a relatively new manufacturing technique (Bozard, n.d.). With this idea comes the dispute of whether it is viable for new technologies to replace older ones. Currently, stamping is still a relatively traditional manufacturing technique which is used to manufacture parts across various industries. 3D printing, on the other hand, has not yet been completely standardized in the manufacturing industry and as of now, its initial costs are still too high for it to be standardized. However, as it becomes more popular and widespread, the production of 3D printers will increase while its cost will continually decrease.

By considering the advantages and disadvantages of both technologies and determining which manufacturing technique may be better suited towards manufacturing PPE, one may conclude that stamping is ideal for mass manufacturing PPEs of one size. PPEs that are simplistic in design and do not require customization, such as masks for the everyday person, would be more efficiently manufactured by stamping presses, as the duration of construction would be significantly shorter than 3D printing. In contrast, 3D printing is an ideal technique for generating customized PPE. For example, PPEs that are moulded to fit specific faces would be particularly useful for medical personnel and other frontline workers. This is suitable because as aforementioned, 3D printers have lower production costs and take less time to manufacture more complex parts, and they are very easily customizable as well.

Interestingly, 3D printing can actually also be used in conjunction with stamping, as it can be used to print new dies to be used in stamping (Matisons, 2015). This would cut the costs incurred in stamping when attempting to customize products and create new designs, as using 3D printers rather than diemakers would significantly lower the labour costs. Thus, instead of pitting these two industrial techniques against each other, they can be used synergistically to contribute to the success of the final product. However, the main problem existing with this idea is that it is more cost and time effective to use 3D printers alone to produce certain products. Rather than 3D printing several stamping dies to be used in a stamping press, it might be more efficient to simply use the 3D printer itself to generate the desired product.

# Chapter 10

## HYDROFORMING

Hydroforming is a metal fabricating process that is used to alter and change the shape of a metal object (American Hydroformers, n.d.). This molding process is commonly used for metallic materials, such as steel, copper, aluminum, and brass. Currently, there are two different ways in which hydroforming can be done: sheet hydroforming and tube hydroforming (American Hydroformers, n.d.). However, the overall idea of hydroforming is essentially the same for the two methods. Both of these techniques use dies, which are essentially the "molds" of the desired shape, and they both involve the pumping of high-pressure water. The purpose of this water is to apply a pressure on the metal to change its shape, hence the name, hydroforming (American Hydroformers, n.d.). However, depending on the specific process, the location where the high-pressure water is pumped may vary. The image below displays the simplified step by step process of tube hydroforming.

Tube hydroforming uses half-dies to alter the metal into the desired shape (Jones Metal Products [JMP], 2017). The two ends of the pipes allow for the high-pressure hydraulic fluids to flow through the metal and cause the material to expand (JMP, 2017). The dies surrounding the pipe then ensure that this expansion results in the desired shape. Once this desired form is reached, the fluid is then emptied from the metal and the metal is removed (JMP, 2017).

When tube hydroforming a metal, it is important to consider the shape of the initial material. If the starting metal has bends and curves, the material would first need to undergo the process of tube bender (American Hydroformer, n.d.). In this process, the metal is placed under a pre-form press where pressure is applied to the metal to remove the bends (American Hydroformer, n.d.). Afterwards, the hydroforming process is then applied to the metal to obtain the desired shape. Once this shape has formed, there may be further steps, such as laser cutting, to make the shape as precise as possible (American Hydroformer, n.d.). This type of hydroforming can be used to create car frames, brass tubes for instruments and aluminum bicycle frames. The other form of hydroforming is sheet hydroforming, which uses one die instead of the two used in tube hydroforming. In this case, a sheet of metal is placed on top of the die and instead of having a second die that would go on top, a blank holder plate would occupy this space instead (JMP, 2017). This blank holder plate is created with an injection channel in the middle which allows for the hydraulic fluid to flow through. In this case the pressure of the hydraulic fluid causes the sheet metal to bend towards and in the shape of the die.

Although sheet hydroforming is commonly used to create curved metal form sheet metals, it also has the capability to create many other geometric shapes from a large variety of metals, such as aluminum, steel, titanium, and many more (JMP, 2017). Due to its ability to create complex shapes, it is often used in many industries, such as healthcare, aerospace, and commercial lighting (JMP, 2017). The parts created by this process can be used as covers for equipment or for parts to make that equipment that are in need of protection (JMP, 2017).

In relation to additive manufacturing, 3D printing can be particularly useful in the hydroforming process. One of the ways in which 3D printing may be involved is the manufacturing of the various components used in the hydroforming process. In many cases, the parts needed for hydroforming can be difficult to gather and put together. In particular, the creation of the die molds can be remarkably difficult and time consuming as many of these die molds are manufactured separately (Ahmetoglu, 2001). However, through the 3D printing technique of fused deposition modeling, the pipes, dies and blank holders that are needed for the hydroforming process can be easily created (Proto3000, n.d.). This can minimize the amount of time spent on setting-up the machine and allow for production to begin much sooner. Additionally, 3D printing techniques may also be integrated into other aspects of the hydroforming process to improve the overall efficiency. For instance, 3D printing can be utilized during the planning phase of hydroforming. Essentially, this translates to creating a 3D printed scale model of the final product. By examining this inexpensive and quickly assembled model, manufacturers would be able to determine the most appropriate hydroforming approach, thereby reducing the time and costs involved with the decision-making process (JMP, 2015).

Since it is clear that 3D printing technology can be used to complement hydroforming processes, the increased efficiency of the overall process can be particularly useful during a pandemic setting. With speed being one of the most important advantages during a crisis, this optimized process can allow for a faster response by manufacturers. However, with the context of the PPE shortage, hydroforming may not be particularly useful as it can only be done with metals Since the PPEs used in hospitals are not composed of metal, this form of manufacturing cannot be used. Despite this, however, this combination of 3D printing and hydroforming can still play a major role during the COVID-19 pandemic as metal parts are commonly used in medical instruments and devices (Fluid Forming Americas, n.d.). With the effects of this pandemic extending beyond the realm of PPEs, it is important to ensure that there are sufficient amounts of other types of medical equipment. For this reason, despite hydroforming being unable to produce the desperately needed PPEs, this manufacturing technique can still support the fight against COVID-19 by supplying workers with other types of crucially important equipment.

Since the importance of hydroforming was established in the previous paragraph, it is crucial to understand the advantages and disadvantages of this technology. Beginning with the advantages, part consolidation is one of the benefits of hydroforming. Part consolidation refers to the idea of being able to produce an entire product at once without having to produce multiple parts that would be put together later on. This ability is very advantageous as it would require much more time to consolidate all the separate parts. Without this step, the final product can be produced in roughly 20 seconds after it is loaded into the hydroforming machine (Ahmetoglu, 2001).

Another benefit of hydroforming is that it can cost effectively create strong structures. In many cases, the thickness of the product is important in order to ensure that the metal does not bend. However, if the wall of the product is too thick then the weight would increase, thereby making the production much more expensive (JMP, 2015). Fortunately, through a well-designed process, hydroforming is capable of manufacturing products that can withstand high pressure and not bend. Hydroforming can also ensure that the final product is of the desired thickness and with a reduced weight (JMP, 2015). This makes hydroforming a very powerful and efficient process as strong and inexpensive products are commonly required by customers.

Regarding the precision of the hydroforming process, further improvements in area depend on the advancements of other technologies. This is evident with the development of a new hydroforming technique that allows the material to be accurately reformed into a well-designed shape. This newly added process is controlled by a computer which allows for the material to undergo high pressure, thereby causing it to form into the desired shape (American Hydroformer, 2014). Therefore, the accuracy of hydroforming is a developing area of research and further advancements in this technology may depend on the improvements of other STEM fields. For now, however, hydroforming offers tight dimensional tolerance, meaning that the dimensions are precisely exact and there are very few errors in the production through this method (Ahmetoglu, 2001). Interesting, the technology used in this production also allows for low spring back (Ahmetoglu, 2001). This is especially important in the car industry as low spring back allows there to be safety for the car when it encounters objects, such as speed bumps. Furthermore, hydroforming is also a relatively resourceful technique as it is capable of reusing material. Accidentally bent or broken parts of the material can be shaped into the product by repeating the hydroforming process, thereby minimizing the amount of wasted material (American Hydroformer, 2014). Finally, the last advantage that will be discussed is hydroforming's ability to form complex shapes from the metal material. Since the process of hydroforming is capable of forming a large variety of shapes, this presents designers with a substantial amount of designer freedom (American Hydroformers, 2014).

While it is clear that hydroforming is an effective and advantageous technique, there are many disadvantages as well. For instance, the equipment required for the hydroforming process are not only expensive, but also require a long time to produce (Ahmetoglu, 2001). This can be particularly disadvantageous during a pandemic setting as time is of the essence. Another disadvantage is that the equipment for one hydroforming process can only be used to form one type of object due to the molds that are being used (Ahmetoglu, 2001). Therefore, it would be remarkably expensive and time-consuming to purchase the equipment for customized objects. Thus, the products being produced are commonly mass manufactured to make this process economically feasible. Lastly, another limitation for the process of hydroforming is that the only material that can be used are metals. As previously mentioned, in the case of PPEs, metals are rarely used and thus the process of hydroforming cannot be used (Ahmetoglu, 2001).

Evidently, hydroforming is a remarkably important metal fabrication process that has a variety of uses in the industrial field. From supplying healthcare facilities with medical equipment to producing automotive parts, hydroforming has a large range of potential applications in modern society. Fortunately, with the development of 3D printing, this process can be further optimized and operate much more efficiently. Although this process may be unable to produce PPEs during this severe international shortage, hydroforming is not useless as it continues to support the healthcare system by producing other types of crucially important medical equipment and devices.

# Chapter 11

## 3D PRINTED MASKS

In the midst of a global pandemic, preventive measures as simple as wearing masks in communal places can help stop the spread of COVID-19. Governments, workplaces and institutions around the world have implemented the usage of face masks for the collective communities' safety, as masks have been scientifically proven to limit the transmission of viral respiratory droplets.

Recently, several local and federal governments have enforced laws making it compulsory for all individuals to wear face masks when in public spaces. Even when not in public, avoiding touching the face and only using clean hands around the face is recommended at all times. Additionally, it is advised to never touch the outer surface of the masks with bare hands, as it may be contaminated with virus particles. The following recommendations have been made by healthcare professionals to ensure face masks are worn and used correctly: fit the mask tightly across the bridge of the nose and the mouth without leaving  any gaps to prevent particle transmission and infection, pull the mask to the bottom of the chin and ensure that it covers most of the face as a protective barrier (Peek, 2020). Depending on the number of times worn and duration, surgical masks and N95 respirators can be reused, but the dampness of the inner surface is an indication that the mask must be changed according to the World Health Organization (World Health Organization [WHO], 2020a). When storing masks for later use, isolating masks in plastic or paper bags for two to three days is scientifically recommended (Peek, 2020). Cloth masks can be washed and reused on a regular basis and in recent times, people have been layering cloth masks on top of surgical masks in order to increase the longevity of surgical masks or N95 respirators, which can be relatively expensive (Peek, 2020) Cloth masks are quite easy to wash in regular laundry machines and by hand as well.

Moreover, critical questions regarding feasibility, wearability and accessibility arise when determining and comparing the effectiveness of different groups of masks. To elaborate, surgical masks are designed to be disposable and relatively fitted, to prevent the wearer from spreading large droplet particles from a cough or sneeze (Peek, 2020). However, surgical masks are very permeable, thus they are unable to provide protection against viral particles (Peek, 2020). On the other hand, N95 respirators are more tightly and properly fitted to the face than surgical masks (Peek, 2020). In addition, they are tested to block both smaller particles as well as large droplets to minimize the risk of COVID-19 infection. While surgical masks are more easily accessible and can be worn for longer periods of time without discomfort, N95 respirators are less permeable than surgical masks, thus they are designed for medical professionals in the frontlines and have a limited supply (Peek, 2020). Cloth masks can also act as somewhat of a barrier to large droplets (Peek, 2020). However, as they offer much less protection than surgical masks and N95 respirators, only everyday individuals are recommended to wear them (not medical personnel). Depending on the number of layers worn behind the cloth mask, it is possible for cloth masks to prevent the transmission by controlling the source. The biggest advantage to cloth masks is that they are widely available for public usage and fashion-forward.

Mask efficacy and protection has been an ongoing debate since the beginning of the pandemic. Scientific studies have shown that the direct transmission of airborne droplets is limited by surgical masks and N95 respirators (Worby & Chang, 2020). Approximately 80% of small particles and 96% of pathogens are blocked out by surgical masks, providing three times more protection than regular cloth face coverings. In influenza studies, clustered random trials have shown that one's likelihood of exposure to the virus and transmission are greatly decreased with the usage of face masks and regular hand washing (Worby & Chang, 2020). For N95 respirators, studies have shown that they are able to filter out 95% of 0.3-micrometer airborne particles (Ishack & Lipner, 2020). Thus, they are effective at restricting not only droplets but airborne particles as well. However, since the wearing of masks has been recommended by various institutions, government officials, and international organizations, many myths and controversies have arisen regarding masks. Protestors have claimed that masks are the cause for hyperventilating, hypoxia and many other medical conditions without sufficient medical evidence. According to the WHO, although wearing masks for a long period of time can cause discomfort, there are no signs that they cause oxygen deficiency or carbon dioxide intoxication (WHO, 2020a).

The diminishing supply of face masks has been a global crisis since the start of the pandemic, due to the rate at which they are being used up. Although the masks deemed acceptable by governments and medical professionals include cloth masks, surgical masks and respirators like N95 masks, many began to use scarves and plastic bags as a face covering amidst the large mask shortages. The supply and demand model of face masks have shown that their demand is much higher than their supply. The supply of masks available for frontline workers has been depleting due to rising COVID-19 cases, thus all healthcare institutions have a high demand for masks (Peek, 2020). Masks are in large demand by common individuals as well due to the widespread fear of the coronavirus. Panic buying has caused shortages and to mitigate such effects, the Taiwanese government has imposed limits on the number of masks that their citizens can buy per week in their national health cards as a coping strategy to keep up with the rate of depletion of the supplies (Peek, 2020). Namely, being able to deploy supplies when necessary and allocate resources to healthcare industries and individuals in high risk institutions such as prisons and senior homes have been a priority for many countries. The restrictions and obligations regarding wearing face masks remain blurry in some areas including some regions in Canada, where initiatives like social distancing can arguably reduce the need for masks.

The mass production of 3D printed masks is an avenue by which the shortages of Personal Protective Equipment (PPE) can be addressed. 3D printed masks allow for mass manufacturing in order to meet the high demand of masks across the globe. An advantage of 3D printed masks is that they can be personalized to fit the face of an individual instead of a one-size product for all users - this idea of customizability will be discussed more in detail in a later chapter. During the COVID-19 pandemic, the Imperial College London began to move the materials and resources that were previously used for sleep apnea studies to a workspace that researches and produces 3D printed masks (British Broadcasting Corporation (BBC), 2020). In this initiative, custom fitted masks and respirators are being created using a face scan, followed by a few forms which must be filled out on their website and lastly printed by the Autodesk 360 platform (British Broadcasting Corporation (BBC), 2020). There are other institutions as well, like the Barrow Neurological Institute, who have successfully 3D printed N95 respirators and gave open access of 3D printer design files and assembly instructions to the public, which encouraged people with personal 3D printers at home to print the given PPE designs and possibly help their own family, community or local healthcare institutions (British Broadcasting Corporation (BBC), 2020). At Barrow, they have used FDM printers to print these PPE due to their efficiency and reliability, but all open-access files created are compatible with any 3D printer (British Broadcasting Corporation (BBC), 2020). For credibility purposes, their filters on the N95 respirators mirror the 3M P100 filters and are certified by the National Institute for Occupational Safety and Health with an emergency use permission from the United States Food and Drug Administration (FDA) (British Broadcasting Corporation [BBC], 2020). In another study, Swennen, Pottel and Haers (2020) have demonstrated a proof of concept (PoC) for the effectiveness of 3D printed face masks with global accessibility but cautions all users to receive official authorization for public use by their local authorities. In essence, the design process uses Computer-Aided Design (CAD) software and reusable templates to create printing instructions. Boolean calculations are then computed, and face scans are taken to generate a durable and effective 3D printed face mask (Swennen et al., 2020). A 3D printing company demonstrated the easy global accessibility of 3D printed face masks through PoC by contributing more designs.

The 3D printing process initially begins with a CAD file which provides the design and instructions for the mask, subsequently followed by the printing itself via 3D printers (Barrow Neurological Institution, 2020). The main components of the mask include the 3D printed solid face covering, the disposable straps and the filter membrane (Barrow Neurological Institution, 2020). It may be important to acknowledge that individuals may have allergies to the materials used to create both the disposable and non-disposable parts of the printed masks (Barrow Neurological Institution, 2020). After the mask has been printed, it is outlined with clay on the lining of the inner side, followed by the repair of any additional leaks. After these steps have been completed, the clay is then heated (Barrow Neurological Institution, 2020). The usage of clay is what allows the shape and size of the mask to be customizable for different individuals. Following this, a silicon mould is created around the masks and is cured with great precision (Barrow Neurological Institution, 2020). An optional step of a PLA seam can be added between the coupler and the mask. Lastly, any choice of straps is attached to complete the 3D printed product (Barrow Neurological Institution, 2020).

In addition to being commonly utilized in the making of 3D printed masks, face scanning technology is also commonly used in facial plastic surgery and craniofacial surgery.With the addition of form fitting, 3D facial scanning enables 3D printed products to be customized to each individual. Furthermore, the face scanning technology works without actually coming into contact with a given individual, which is a major advantage during this pandemic as it enables social distancing and minimizes one's risk of infection during face scanning. Face scanning can also be done using a phone application, such as the Bellus3D application (Barrow Neurological Institution; Ishack & Lipner, 2020). The greatest advantages of this face scanning technology are the anthropometric graphics of facial features including facial hair size and density, which can allow the printer to develop masks with a better seal and fit (Ishack & Lipner, 2020). In a study which examined the seal of 3D printed N95 masks, the prototypes which used Acrylonitrile Butadiene Styrene plastic and were printed from a Fused Deposition Modeling (FDM) 3D printer showed better results in terms of fit and seal than 3M 8210 N95 FFR respirator masks (Ishack & Lipner, 2020).

To delve deeper, as mentioned in previous chapters, there is a range of 3D printers such as FDM, SLS and many others which are accessible in many industries, and these printers are able to be mass manufactured at a relatively low cost. The components and materials used for filters, straps and raw materials in 3D printing can be easily found in various places across the globe – the straps are made of elastic bands or Velcro and the filters can be easily constructed from industrial fabrics. These printers and materials can produce both 3D printed masks and 3D printed respirators, which may be as effective as certified surgical and N95 respirators which were manufactured using conventional methods (Ishack & Lipner, 2020). Furthermore, the standard filtration material for N95 respirators consists of polypropylene (PP) with a partial crystalline structure (Ishack & Lipner, 2020). However, recently it has been suggested that a blend of PP and styrene-(ethylene-butylene)-styrene (SEBS) is more effective, which is recommended for 3D printing N-95 respirators as it is able to withstand higher temperature conditions during the printing process (Ishack & Lipner, 2020). This mixture also allows durability to last for a longer period of time, as well as more flexibility under different conditions such as during possible sterilization or disinfection of the respirator. Depending on the type and the duration of use, filters used for 3D printed respirators can be also obtained from trusted vendors who offer better protection and circulation.

Although many advantages of 3D printing masks have been discussed, it is also important to caution all people that in order to use 3D printed masks, they require clinical testing and proper authorization from the government or health and safety institutions. Currently, many governments have temporarily authorized the use of 3D printed masks in this pandemic in order to combat widespread shortages (Swennen et al., 2020). However, as printed masks have not been authorized or officially certified by the government or health organizations for the long-term, many hospitals still prefer to use PPE from known and trusted companies. Whether printed masks can be reused or cleaned by disinfection is also another point of concern during PPE shortages, as layer lines from the 3D printer may prevent the masks from being able to be fully sanitized ("The Problems with 3D Printed Respirator", 2020). Hence, it is also argued that for safety reasons, they will have to be disposable until there is a better way to disinfect the masks. In the case of sterilization or disinfection and the presence of high temperatures, the durability of 3D printed masks should also be tested to ensure mask durability in these conditions for health and safety reasons, as this will vary from one manufacturer to another ("The Problems with 3D Printed Respirator", 2020). Depending on the design, materials, and manufacturing company, the mask may not be exactly form fitting. If 3D printing manufacturers use rigid materials or if their designs have flaws, the crevasses in the masks may not be sealed and thus masks may not be accurately fitted to an individual's face ("The Problems with 3D Printed Respirator", 2020). According to some skeptics of 3D printed PPE, 3D masks should be used as a last resort when all other supply options have been exhausted instead of mobilizing printers to create thousands and thousands of 3D printed masks ("The Problems with 3D Printed Respirator", 2020).

To end, masks have long been used to protect the public against droplets and viral particles, ever since the influenza outbreak in 1918 (Little, 2020). During World War I, mask wearing was as important as wartime duty and some actually considered it deadlier than the war itself (Little, 2020). People in the 21st century have access to an unthinkable amount of technology to improve and innovate the realm of mask making. With the world population at an all-time high, 3D printed masks which offer a lower cost and customized fit is an attractive option for both developed and developing countries to prevent the transmission of COVID-19. With a great selection of materials, printers, protection and price range to choose from, many institutions can benefit from this useful technology during the pandemic. Whether masks are only being printed because of shortages, for one's personal protection, or to provide an upgrade from regular masks in terms of fit and cost efficiency, many studies have demonstrated the efficiency of 3D printed masks and respirators in limiting the spread of the virus. Therefore, with proper authorization from official institutions, making use of this technology is highly recommended to tackle widespread pandemic equipment shortages.

# Chapter 12

## N95 RESPIRATORS AND MASKS WITH VISORS

N95 respirators are another form of personal protective equipment (PPE) which have been used frequently during the pandemic are another form of personal protective equipment (PPE) which have been used frequently during the pandemic. Their design allows for a close facial fit which in turn allows for highly efficient airborne particle filtration. The respirator is designed to create an effective seal around the nose and mouth, which is why it is fitted tightly to the face (U.S. Food and Drug Administration [FDA], 2020c). Surgical N95 respirators are commonly used in the healthcare field and are deemed essential supplies for healthcare workers to prevent the spread of viral droplets and airborne virus particles. Additionally, these respirators must undergo various rounds of testing for many factors due to their extensive role in protecting frontline medical personnel. These tests include filtration efficiency (particulate and bacterial), fluid resistance, flammability, and biocompatibility (FDA, 2020c). Sharing and/or reusing N95 respirators is highly discouraged as it is possible for the respirator to become contaminated in its first use, thus sharing or reusing it could potentially spread the virus and cause infection. This is especially true in the healthcare field as healthcare workers treating patients with COVID-19 are highly likely to be exposed to dangerous contaminants, however this exposure could be limited by the proper usage of these respirators. For regular users of N95 respirators, it should be noted that if it becomes harder to breathe when wearing a respirator, it should be replaced with a new one. In order to dispose of the damaged mask correctly, it should be placed in a medical waste bag and hands should be washed immediately after the mask has been discarded. There are some precautions that should be taken before wearing these masks. It is important to check with a family doctor about whether it is suitable to use N95 respirators as they can make it more difficult to breathe. This applies to people with pre-existing chronic respiratory illnesses or any other related medical condition related to difficulties in breathing (FDA, 2020c). Furthermore, to target the issue of breathability, many N95 respirator masks come with an exhalation valve that is used to reduce heat buildup and to make it easier for the wearer to breathe (FDA, 2020c). Additionally, as N95 respirators are designed to be fitted to the face, this mask typically cannot be worn by children or people with facial hair as this mask was not designed to fit their specific facial features; thus, the masks are not able to provide protection to their fullest extent.

With the onset of the COVID-19 pandemic, N95 respirators became a very commonly used PPE, especially by healthcare professionals, as a means of protection. Due to the pandemic, there have been new guidelines set for the reuse and decontamination of the respirator. The following guidelines have been set by the FDA and are prone to changes and edits due to the developing situation with the COVID-19 pandemic. As a result of the large shortages of PPE across the globe, often healthcare personnel are left with no choice but to reuse these masks and therefore new temporary guidelines have ensued which allow for the decontamination and reuse of these masks. However, it has been recommended that when available, new masks should be used at all times; used masks that have been decontaminated should only be used as a last resort. The N95 respirators that have exhalation valves, however, are not to go through the decontamination process, as these valves can break down when subject to sterilization (FDA, 2020c). In order to ensure adequate sterilization and safe use, the decontamination process has to be approved by the National Institute for Occupational Safety and Health, and the Food and Drug Administration has provided an evaluation system for proper decontamination technique (FDA, 2020c).

In terms of efficiency, the N95 respirator is proven to be more efficient than the surgical mask as it has the ability to filter both small airborne particles and larger droplets. The N95 respirator is designed to block and filter 95% of all small particles present in one's environment (FDA, 2020c). Research shows that N95 respirators' efficiency increases with the size of the particle; meaning that the bigger the particle, the easier it is for it to be blocked by the mask (Qian et al., 1998). To use the N95 mask, healthcare providers must be trained to ensure proper wearing and usage of the mask, and they must pass a test before being able to use it in the workplace. One of the important issues surrounding some N95 respirators is that the exhalation valve, while improving breathability, does not prevent other people around the wearer from becoming infected if the wearer does have an airborne infectious disease. Due to the chance of the spread of virus through the exhalation valve, many places have banned the N95 masks with these valves.

In recent times, as the virus continued to spread globally, the shortage of N95 masks began to put pressure on healthcare providers and the government. As mentioned in past chapters, Canada's shortage became larger with the United States' President Trump ordering 3M, a company known for its production of N95 respirators, to stop shipping to Canada. With the pre-existing widespread shortages exacerbated by export restrictions, Canada and various other countries have been seeking alternative sources and production methods to meet the growing demand of N95 respirators. As 3D printing has emerged as a new, efficient manufacturing method in recent times, many have turned to this technology to produce PPE and to help alleviate the burden felt by the healthcare community due to this shortage. During the pandemic, there has been a lot of progress regarding 3D printing N95 respirator replacements. These replacements, produced with 3D printers, have been shown to have the same impact and efficiency as N95 respirators (Barrow Neurological Institution, 2020). One example of a company that produces these replacement masks is Copper 3D which uses nanotechnology and 3D printing to produce reusable plastic N95 respirators (Copper 3D, 2020). Another institute that takes part in creating replacement N95 respirators is the Barrow Neurological Institute, as mentioned in the previous chapter (Barrow Neurological Institution, 2020). The president, Michael T. Lawton, has 3D printed an N95 respirator replacement using different materials such as a silicone part which allows the 3D printed mask to be fitted onto the patients faces, thus allowing for a fitted seal to be formed as well as effective sizing (Barrow Neurological Institution, 2020). Using a P100 mask allows for better filtration, and it is also a safer option in comparison to the N95 mask (Barrow Neurological Institution, 2020). In comparison to N95 masks, P100 masks are oil proof and protect the wearer against a higher percentage of particles, more specifically 99.8% of particles (Barrow Neurological Institution, 2020). As discussed, it is clear that the N95 respirator 3D printed replacements are a better choice in terms of efficiency in terms of their customization and being able to provide a much better protection. However, as 3D printing is still a relatively new technology which can take a relatively longer amount of time to produce parts, these replacements are not affordable for everyone and most definitely not accessible to everyone in the healthcare community yet.

Another form of personal protective equipment that is becoming increasingly popular in the public is face shields and masks with visors (Gray, 2020). They consist of a band that goes around the head which is attached to a that provides a barrier for the face from the surroundings. At the beginning of the pandemic, face shields were mostly used amongst individuals in manufacturing industries (Gray 2020). Now, as of August 2020, face shields are also commonly used in restaurants, salons, and spas (Gray, 2020). They seem to extend the usefulness of face masks as they cover the entire face, not only from the front but also from the sides. Typically, face masks or respirators are worn on the face underneath the face shield in order to maximize the protection provided by both of these PPE (Gray, 2020). Face shields, as with many other PPE, are very high in demand during the pandemic due to their protective qualities. It is important to note that the medical community in particular is in need of these products in order to protect themselves, as they encounter patients with the virus every day. Due to the high demand of this product, many manufacturers have mobilized their available resources and have been using them to mass produce face shields.

As mentioned above, the two important parts of face shields/visors are: the lens plate (the shield) and the visors and the strap. The lens plate needs to be made of a material that allows for visual clarity and durability (Thomasnet, 2020). The material that is most commonly used to produce lens plates is polycarbonate, however often other materials such as polyester are used due to their low cost (Thomasnet, 2020). Regardless of the material used, the lens plate must be rigid enough to withstand a substantial amount of pressure and it must protect the wearer from coming into contact with respiratory droplets and other hazardous liquids. Furthermore, the visors and the straps for these face shields are commonly made by injection molding manufacturing processes. During the production process, manufacturers must ensure that the visors and the straps allow for size adjustment and that they are durable enough to last throughout all of the long hours worked by members of the medical community (Gray, 2020). In order to ensure durability, for the medical community, the manufacturers produce visors and straps made of foam that can be adjusted and can hold up the lens plate. In general, face shields are easily disposable and inexpensive due to their light weight, which is beneficial for healthcare providers as disposable PPE ensures that no contaminants are being transferred. The company Sailworks reportedly takes 50 hours to produce 500 face shields from the time that the demand is received (Thomasnet, 2020). However, as the pandemic has dramatically increased the demand for PPE, these shields are now mass produced, yielding about 400 to 500 face shields per day (Thomasnet, 2020).

Undoubtedly, face shields are highly effective forms of PPE, in addition to face masks. However, there has been an enormous shortage of PPE during this pandemic. As workers in the healthcare field have been under immense pressure with insufficient supply, reusing masks has become much more common. Evidently, this is not an ideal situation as disposing of PPE after each use is much safer, thus medical workers usually reuse face shields to extend the amount of time that the face masks worn underneath the visor can last. With the lens plate over the mask, the mask underneath can last longer as the lens plate is providing an extra layer of protection (Mundell, 2020). Although the effectiveness of each of these PPE individually has been demonstrated, this proves that face shields and visors, when used in combination, can be extremely efficient during crises like these in the medical field. In the public, however, usually face visors and shields are worn without masks underneath and even in this case, they have been proven to offer more protection than cloth face masks (Mundell, 2020). The protective ability of the face visor is very dependent on its design and whether it covers the entire face, including the ears and from the forehead to below the chin. One of the many advantages of face shields and visors is the ability to reuse the lens plates with sterilization (Mundell, 2020). In addition to this,as they cover the entire face, face shields and visors prevent the wearer from touching their face and are much more comfortable to wear than masks due to easier breathability.

Finally, with 3D printing face shields and visors, the parts are printed individually and later assembled. The parts are the lens plate, the strap, and the visor, however in many cases it is much easier to use foam as a visor since it is more comfortable and durable, which is more effective for the purposes of the medical community. The visor can be printed from PLA (polylactic acid) or from PETG (Polyethylene terephthalate glycol) (Simplify3D, 2020). If the face shields are to be sterilized between uses and reused, PETG is the preferred material as it offers more durability (Simplify3D, 2020). The production of the lens plate is more complicated in the sense that it is dependent on the situation and case that the face shield is being used for. If the maker is preparing to mass manufacture the lens plates, the ideal material used would be polycarbonate (Simplify3D, 2020). On the other hand, many use 3D printing technologies for their ability to customize PPE and in the case of printing lens plates, PETG is the most common material used. This is due to the various different types of 3D printers that exist and the different settings and skills that are needed to operate certain printers. One must know what material would be ideal and bend correctly, which varies depending on the 3D printing technique being used and whether the manufacturer desires to create customized face shields or mass manufactured face shields Other materials that could be used to 3D print lens plates include propionate, acetate, and polyvinyl chloride (Simplify3D, 2020). One thing that should be done once the parts are printed is to test the flexibility of the visors to make sure that they can be adjusted if required. Additionally, disinfection is also an important step to take when 3D printing face shields. This can be done through placing the product into bleach for a short amount of time after printing to ensure sanitation. As face shields have been proven to provide effective protection against droplets, they are evidently an effective form of PPE. Furthermore, they are very suitable for 3D printing considering the few parts that are needed to create a face shield, as well as the wide availability of plastic materials used in manufacturing. It should be noted, however, that it may take a longer period of time for the product to be printed in comparison to traditional mass manufacturing methods. Additionally, the 3D printed face shield could end up being expensive for the buyer or the one providing the material as more customization is needed and thus more money is spent on this process.

# Chapter 13

## HAZMAT SUITS & GLOVES

As mentioned in previous chapters, upon the onset of the COVID-19 pandemic, public health systems globally implemented policies mandating the use of PPE. Specifically, the two PPEs that will be discussed in this chapter are hazmat suits and gloves. Hazmat suits, also known as hazardous material suits, are impermeable full body garments which protect the wearer from injurious materials and substances, such as chemicals and biological agents (Saul, 2014). These suits are commonly worn by people in various professions such as firefighters, paramedics, and chemical spill personnel (Saul, 2014). In the context of COVID-19, however, hazmat suits are predominantly being worn by front-line healthcare workers treating patients with COVID-19 to protect themselves from being exposed to the virus. Front-line healthcare workers also wear medical gloves as PPE, as these specialized gloves also act as a barrier to protect both the wearer and the patient from spreading the disease (Health Canada, 2020b).

Different countries use different methods to categorize the types of hazmat suits. In the United States, they are classified via letters A to D, ranging from the most to least protective (Safety & Health Practitioner [SHP], 2015). Level A suits are vapour-tight, high protection suits which provide a barrier against airborne particles, vapours, gases, mists and splashes. A device called a self-contained breathing apparatus (SCBA) is typically worn inside the suit as well, which is a device worn to provide breathability in an environment in which inhaling the air may be dangerous to one's health (SHP, 2015). Level A hazmat suits are especially crucial to wear when there is a possible threat to the worker's life or health, thus front-line health workers typically wear this kind of suit when coming into contact with an infected patient. Level B suits protect the wearer against hazardous liquids, but do not offer protection against vapours. Level C suits are also splash-protectant and provide some protection against chemicals and airborne substances, but not enough protection for chemical emergencies. Finally, level D suits do not provide any protection against chemicals; no respirator is worn with these suits either (SHP, 2015).

While hazmat suits are designed to be as impermeable as possible while maintaining breathability, these PPEs still have their disadvantages. Heat stress, for instance, is a common drawback associated with these suits – being clothed in an airtight chemical protective garment causes a heat chamber to be created inside the suit (Milford, 2014). This causes considerable discomfort for medical workers who are required to wear these suits for hours on end. However, it should be noted that manufacturers are actively working on attempting to design more breathable and comfortable suits (Milford, 2014). Another major disadvantage of hazmat suits is the process of removing them, which, in itself, can prove to be a very difficult and meticulous process. If the suit is not removed with caution, it can actually contaminate the wearer – when the hazmat suit is exposed to biohazards, the wearer must ensure they do not come into contact with the outside of the suit, or they must decontaminate the external part of the suit entirely to ensure safety. Contamination during careless removal is quite common and has actually caused numerous medical worker deaths during the Ebola outbreak, thus public health agencies advise against anyone, but medical professionals with proper training from wearing these suits (Kale, 2020). In fact, everyday people wearing hazmat suits to protect themselves against coronavirus can actually cause more harm and contamination than good due to the likelihood of improper removal (Christian, 2020).

Globally, DuPont is the leading company that manufactures the most hazmat suits every year (Milford, 2014). The company uses a trademarked synthetic fabric which is used in hazmat suits and other protective garments, known as Tyvek. This fabric is spun from high density fibers of polyethylene (DuPont Tyvek, n.d.), which is a common thermoplastic used globally. Specifically, for medical hazmat suits, DuPont uses a fabric sub-brand of Tyvek known as Tychem, which is made up of several barrier layers to protect against biohazards like viruses (DuPont, n.d.). DuPont manufactures a variety of hazmat suits offering different levels of protection at numerous costs, ranging from $5 up to over $1,000 (Mody & Manning, 2020). According to the United Nations Office for the Coordination of Humanitarian Affairs (OCHA), the average cost of a hazmat suit is approximately $61.48 USD (Birks, 2014), however, the surge in demand amidst the outbreak of the coronavirus has caused the prices of hazmat suits, and all PPE in general, to skyrocket (Diaz et al., 2020), causing shortages and leaving companies like DuPont scrambling to increase production. In order to meet this rise in demand, in April of 2020, DuPont began doubling its output of protective garments made per month, from 15 million to 30 million (Jain & Nair, 2020). As a result of having to increase PPE production during other viral outbreaks, such as the Ebola virus, DuPont has been able to increase its agility in supply operations during the COVID-19 outbreak (Mody & Manning, 2020). Other large hazmat suit manufacturers include 3M Company, Honeywell Inc., and Ansell Inc (Thomas Industry, n.d.). As hazmat suits are made to protect one's life against biohazards, their manufacturing is an extremely thorough and painstaking process – each suit is handmade, and they are inspected by machines and manually before getting shipped (Kale, 2020).

While 3D printing is currently being used as a means to manufacture several PPEs in order to provide an alternate supply for diminishing PPE globally, medical hazmat suits are not a PPE that is being 3D printed. As aforementioned, Tychem is the primary fabric which is used in hazmat suits protecting against viruses (Rhodes, 2015), however Tychem is currently not compatible with 3D printers. Currently, 3D printers most commonly use plastic, however they are also able to print a large assortment of other materials including metals, nylon, wood, ceramics, wax, paper, sandstone, and photopolymers (von Übel, 2019). In addition, 3D printers are compatible with various composites of the aforementioned materials, such as alumide, which is a nylon-aluminum hybrid (von Übel, 2019). It is possible that as the 3D printing industry expands, manufacturers may innovate their printers to print Tychem products, or potentially develop a new impermeable composite material.

Besides this, there are a plethora of regulations and restrictions placed on the manufacturing of hazmat suits. As these suits are integral to protecting the lives of healthcare workers, they must be designed to be completely impermeable against chemical and biological hazards. A manufacturer cannot afford to make errors or leave pores in these garments without compromising the wearer's safety. Since 3D printing is a relatively new technology, any printable hazmat suit designs being considered must undergo critical clinical assessment. Additionally, getting a license to produce a hazmat suit is a very expensive and tedious process. According to a spokesperson for PPS, a British manufacturing company, it can often cost £63,000 in order to obtain a certificate to make one suit (Kale, 2020). Being that 3D printing is a relatively new manufacturing technique with many other potential applications that it has yet to explore, it is unlikely that 3D printers will undertake the production of hazmat suits anytime soon.

Next, with the topic of gloves, there is a wide range of different types that can be used in protection against various hazards/contaminants. These include: medical gloves offering protection against biological hazards (made of light latex, vinyl or nitrile, with nitrile providing the highest level of protection against viruses), gloves offering protection against chemical hazards (lighter gloves are made of latex or nitrile while heavier gloves are made of butyl, Viton II, or silver shield), insulated gloves which offer protection against extreme temperatures (terry cloth is used for heat and cryogen is used for cold), and gloves which offer protection against cuts, typically used when working with live animals (made of wire mesh) (University of California, Merced, n.d.). Evidently, for the purposes of protecting oneself from COVID-19, predominantly medical gloves are worn.

Similarly to hazmat suits, medical gloves are designed to provide a barrier so that one can protect their hands from being exposed to infection. Medical gloves may be sterile, meaning that they meet the FDA's standards for sterilization methods, or non-sterile, meaning that are usually not sterilized by the manufacturer, but still must meet the FDA's standard assurance level for sterilization methods (GloveNation, n.d.). A key difference between sterile and non-sterile gloves is their quality and their risk of possessing pinholes – approximately 1.5 to 2.5% of non-sterile gloves in a given sample may have pinholes, while approximately 1.0 to 1.5% of sterile gloves in a given sample may have pinholes (GloveNation, n.d.). Therefore, sterile gloves are more appropriate to wear when performing tasks with high risk of infection, such as surgery or treating a viral patient.

Although medical gloves are designed to protect one's hands and limit their risk of infection and illness, currently the FDA has not approved or authorized any medical gloves which provide specific, impermeable protection against coronavirus (U.S. Food & Drug Administration [FDA], 2020b). Nonetheless, they are still worn by medical personnel treating patients in order to provide a barrier to some extent against the virus. As with hazmat suits, used medical gloves also must be disposed of in the correct manner in order to prevent one from exposing themselves to the contaminants present on the gloves. Any contact made between the skin and the external part of the gloves may result in contamination and subsequent infection, thus it is vital that medical personnel be trained to remove their gloves in the appropriate way. As a result of the fact that there is no guarantee that medical gloves can offer an effective form of protection against COVID-19, and the extreme cautions that must be undertaken during the glove removal process, the Center of Disease Control and Prevention (CDC) actually does not recommend wearing gloves for everyday people as a form of PPE when in public (CDC, 2020b). However, the CDC does recommend that gloves be worn when cleaning and when caring for someone sick. Outside of these two instances, they advise against wearing gloves in public (e.g. gloves are not necessary when touching a shopping cart or using an ATM machine); instead, they recommend washing or sanitizing your hands in order to protect yourself from germs (CDC, 2020b). If the wearing of gloves by everyday people became popularized, it is plausible that many people would consider this extra layer of protection as reason enough to wash their hands less frequently, which may actually do more harm than good.

Medical gloves are typically made using ceramic or aluminum molds, which undergo numerous steps during their manufacturing process (Thomas Industry, 2020). These molds are initially subjected to two treatments (disinfecting using bleach, then coating using calcium nitrate and calcium carbonate), and are then filled with latex, nitrile, or polyvinyl chloride – the longer the material is left on the mold, the thicker the gloves will be. After the desired period of time, the molds are spun to remove excess rubber, rinsed, dried, cured, and rinsed again. Following this, the gloves are rolled and removed from the mold using air jets, thereby completing the production process (Thomas Industry, 2020). Afterwards, gloves must also undergo various rounds of testing, the main test being a regulatory test to determine if the gloves can be used medically. Gloves are screened for pinholes via filling the gloves with water and checking to see for leaks – out of a batch of 100 gloves, if 1.5 or less have leaks, then the gloves are approved for medical grade use. Other subsequent tests performed on the gloves include tests to check for dimensions, a test to check for a specific thickness requirement, sterility tests, tensile and elongation tests, and more (Thomas Industry, 2020).

While the cost of medical gloves varies from company to company, depending on the material, thickness, and several other factors, on average a pack of 100 medical gloves may cost approximately $10 to $20 USD – nearly half of this cost is made up of the cost of raw materials as well as the manufacturing process, while storage costs, factory costs, shipping costs and many others make up the other half (Eagle Protect, 2018). Medical gloves, however, are one of the numerous PPEs whose price has surged during COVID-19 due to an increase in demand. Glove manufacturers, namely Top Glove, Ansell Healthcare, Paul Hartmann AG, Halyard Health, and several others (GlobeNewswire, 2018), have also been rampantly increasing production in recent times in order to meet the shortages of gloves for healthcare professionals.

As a result of the globally emergent PPE shortages during this pandemic, the FDA has issued statements explaining that they will be more flexible with manufacturing regulations (FDA, 2020b). Health Canada has also issued similar statements (Health Canada, 2020c). Although 3D printers have vastly expanded their compatible materials collection to include rubber materials, such as latex and nitrile, the same issue that applied to hazmat suits stands with gloves. As a result of the extensive process that gloves must undergo in order to be approved for medical use, 3D printers are currently not being used to manufacture gloves for COVID-19. Currently, in Canada, the public health system encourages 3D printing manufacturers to obtain certifications to produce Class I medical devices, which include PPE like face shields, N95 respirators, and other medical masks (Zakaib et al., 2020). On the other hand, Class II medical devices and above are products which pose a higher health risk to the patient and/or user; thus they require more extensive certifications. This includes things such as medical exam gloves, oxygen masks, as well as other medical device components (Zakaib et al., 2020). Due to the fact that these devices and PPE protect against more significant biohazards, currently 3D printers are not being used to produce them. For instance, it is crucial for medical gloves to be produced in a manner that minimizes the number of pinholes in order to limit the risk of contamination, which currently cannot be ensured by 3D printers. Therefore, as 3D printing is still a relatively new technology, it is arguable that it is not completely trustworthy. Health Canada does acknowledge, however, that as 3D printing evolves and grows, it may eventually progress to be able to produce Class II medical devices (Health Canada, 2020c) – but as of now, it is not quite there yet.

In summary, hazmat suits and gloves are both integral components of the large assortment of PPEs which help to protect healthcare workers from contracting COVID-19. As both of these PPEs are considered to be Class II or above medical devices, which are considerably more important in preserving the lives of medical personnel, it is essential for these products to be manufactured correctly; virtually without any errors. Consequently, 3D printing has not yet matured enough as a technology and as an industry to be able to manufacture and distribute these types of PPEs. However, as this technology continues to grow rapidly in the medical industry, it is conceivable for 3D printing to expand its range of PPEs. With the way 3D printing has grown exponentially in recent years, the possibilities are limitless!

# Chapter 14

## THE CUSTOMIZATION AND APPLICATIONS OF 3D PRINTING TECHNOLOGY

The exponential surge of COVID-19 cases during this pandemic has been, to say the least, an enormous burden on the healthcare industry. From overworked front-line medical personnel to industrial giants of medical devices and PPE scrambling to respond to the huge shortages, COVID-19 has caused colossal implications for several people and organizations. Amidst the big increases in the mass manufacturing of PPEs, one problem has been significantly overlooked – the importance of customizing PPEs; tailoring them for people who are unable to fit in mass manufactured, one sized garments and equipment.

When there are massive shortages in a product, manufacturing companies are pressured to exponentially increase their output within a very short period of time. As a result, manufacturers opt to increase all factors of production and create as many products in bulk as they can. Therefore, creating customized products of different sizes, materials, fits, etc., would simply take too long and would significantly compromise the ability of manufacturers to promptly meet the needs of hospitals and other institutions in a timely fashion. Thus, companies mass manufacture one-size-fits-all PPEs in order to replenish the rapidly diminishing stock as quickly and effectively as possible. While the mass manufacturing method is theoretically logical, it does not address the specific needs of people, especially minority groups who cannot fit into the one-size PPE being manufactured.

One notable example of a minority group who is negatively affected by this is women – according to British front-line healthcare workers, standardized PPE is leaving female workers unsafe. They claim that "the gear is often designed with male bodies in mind" (Porterfield, 2020), despite the UK Department of Health's statement that the PPE is designed to be unisex (Porterfield, 2020). Intriguingly, many female workers from the National Health Service (NHS) report that the small-est size PPE available for them at work is often too big, in spite of the fact that 77% of NHS workers are women (Porterfield, 2020). They also claim that the coronavi-rus pandemic has exacerbated this problem dramatically. As a result, female NHS workers have stated that they have no choice but to resort to wearing the PPE that is too large for them, often pulling it extremely tight in order to account for the size disparity (Porterfield, 2020). According to the Guardian, some healthcare workers have actually reported developing ulcers and abrasions on their face from pulling ill-fitting masks too tightly (Topping, 2020). Not only does this affect female health workers in the UK, but it reportedly affects females who use PPEs globally during this pandemic (Porterfield, 2020).

Aside from causing extreme discomfort, ill-fitting PPE can actually compromise the safety of healthcare workers and pose life-threatening hazards. Having to wear large, cumbersome masks and face shields can impede on one's sight, which can jeopardize their ability to treat patients (Wilkinson, 2020). If an ill-fitting mask is worn, it often falls down below the nose, and the wearer must constantly adjust it – not only is this an inconvenience for the wearer, but it is a huge health risk, as masks are meant to create a seal and consistently cover both the mouth and nose in order to be deemed effective in preventing the spread of the virus. This is because the mouth and nose, also known as the mucosae, are the main routes of transmission of the virus, thus an ill-fitting mask may leave one route accessible which greatly endangers one's safety (World Health Organization [WHO], 2020e). Furthermore, an oversized mask can fail to create an effective face seal, making the wearer more susceptible to contaminants penetrating through the barrier of the mask and thus becoming infected. The same principle applies to other PPE as well – a medical worker who is meant to wear XXS gloves wearing XXL gloves impairs their dexterity and does not provide an effective seal to prevent contamination (Wilkinson, 2020).

Aside from compromising the lives of healthcare workers who are forced to wear oversized PPE when given no other option during this pandemic, ill-fitting PPE can also endanger the lives of the patients that are being treated by these workers. As ill-fitting PPE does not create an effective seal, workers adorning PPE too large for them are not only more at risk of contracting the virus, but they are also more likely to spread it to patients who may visit the hospital for reasons unrelated to COVID-19. While this may be the reality for women as PPE are often too large for them, it is possible for the same issues to exist with workers who are abnormally large and thus, cannot fit into the limited sizes of PPEs available during the pandemic.

Additionally, besides size, mass manufacturing can possibly pose problems for those who may have allergies to certain materials used in medical equipment. For example, the main materials used to manufacture medical gloves are latex, nitrile, and vinyl, with latex gloves reportedly being frequently used by healthcare workers (Tabary et al., 2020). However, in recent times there have been increasing reports of hypersensitivity to natural rubber latex (NRL) (Tabary et al., 2020). During a time like this where the medical glove shortages are often quite large, it is possible that healthcare workers have no choice but to utilize latex gloves in spite of their allergies or sensitivities. This highlights another problem that exists with mass manufacturing, while simultaneously underlining the importance of PPE customization.

Currently, most PPE is designed to be disposable, as upon the contamination of a PPE, it must be discarded appropriately in order to avoid potentially contaminating other surfaces or individuals. However, as medical personnel must dispose of PPE each time they treat a different patient, it is apparent that the average frontline worker goes through dozens of different protective equipment each day (Johns Hopkins Center for Health Security, 2020). Evidently, the high daily consumption rate of PPE greatly contributes to their widespread shortages across various countries. In addition to this, the massive amounts of PPE being discarded every day during this pandemic generates a significant amount of waste, thus causing harm to the environment as well.

With such a large range of issues involving the traditional manufacturing of PPE, this is where 3D printing comes into play, offering numerous advantages. 3D printing is notorious for offering high customizability in its products; this technology's ability to manufacture complex and highly personalized equipment is unmatched. Face masks can be customized in order to fit the exact parameters of one's face through 3D laser scanning technology. Using this technology, chin arc, jawline, face length, nose length, and nose protrusion measurements can all be taken accurately and virtually instantaneously (Ishack & Lipner, 2020). Thus, this information can be used to manufacture a customized N95 face seal. In addition to ensuring the utmost comfort of the mask wearer, the creation of a personalized seal is very effectively adhered to one's face, thus providing effective protection, which is particularly crucial for medical workers. Although this individualized approach does have its downsides as it requires more time and thus is less efficient to manufacture, it targets issues of personalization that are clearly not met by the conventional mass manufacturing means, as evidenced with the information of NHS workers above.

Furthermore, various members of the global 3D printing community have designed PPE to be reusable in order to target the shortages. However, in order to be deemed effective PPE, they must be adequately sterilized between each use (Tino et al., 2020). Thus, reusable 3D printed PPEs must be disinfected and monitored constantly in order to be used. Additionally, local individuals and institutions must consider whether the sterilization techniques available to them are powerful enough to completely sterilize the reusable PPE – if they are not, the 3D printed equipment likely cannot be used, which is a major drawback of this manufacturing technique (Tino et al., 2020). Currently, the main PPE that is being 3D printed includes: several different designs of medical face masks with reusable filters, reusable respirators, and face shields with a reusable printable headpiece (Tino et al., 2020). Therefore, not only does 3D printing provide the substantial advantage of personalization – fitting the dimensions of PPE to fit a specific individual – but it also prints certain PPE which can be reused. This conserves materials and generates much less waste, in addition to helping reduce the vast shortages – creating reusable PPE through 3D printing lifts some burden off of mass manufacturers who have been frantically generating as much PPE as possible during this pandemic.

With this in mind, 3D printers can act as an alternative source of PPE which caters to individuals' needs, while mass manufacturing techniques can continue to act as a bulk source of PPE to account for the widespread shortages. Additionally, 3D printing is known to be a technology which is able to print complex products more easily than other manufacturing methods – as all designs are created digitally, whether a design is extremely simple or extremely complex, it will likely take nearly the same amount of cost to print both (Rathi, 2018). With other types of manufacturing, additional machines and skills must be utilized in order to create complex parts, thus there is an added cost of assembly (Rathi, 2018). Conversely, 3D printing simply uses an initial digital design and generates the entire part in one process rather than having to create each component individually and assemble it in the end. Therefore, it is sensible to utilize the advantages that 3D printing offers in terms of being able to offer complexity and customizability at no added cost, being that an alternate source (traditional mass manufacturing methods) already exists to print non-personalized PPE.

Besides its application towards generating customized PPE in the context of COVID-19, 3D printing can also be applied to various other areas within the medical field; namely, bioprinting organs and tissues, bioprinting prosthetics and implants, and the delivery and dosage of pharmaceuticals (Nutma, 2019; Ventola, 2014). Currently, the main treatment which exists for organ failure is simply to do an organ transplant from a donor. However, it is well known that there is a huge shortage of donor organs available, thereby resulting in long lists of individuals waiting for organ transplants, which is evidently injurious to their health as their own organs continue to fail. Furthermore, there is a common issue of donor organs or tissues being rejected by an individual's immune system. The new technique of 3D printing organs, while still in its beginning stages, can potentially solve many of these issues. For instance, using one's own stem cells can minimize the risk of tissue rejection, organs can be 3D printed with precise cell placement, and several factors can be controlled by medical professionals, such as the diameter and volume of cells, cell concentration, resolution, speed of printing, etc. (Ventola, 2014). This is very advantageous as specialists and medical personnel can essentially design and print personalized organs for individuals, thereby theoretically maximizing their chance of success. There are, however, several limitations with 3D printing organs as it is still a very new concept. Organs that have been produced thus far are very small and simple – nowhere near the complexity that is needed for the body. Moreover, the printed organs also do not have blood vessels, nerves, or lymph nodes, which are necessary for viable function (Ventola, 2014).

Although organ printing still has a long way to go, 3D printing implants and prostheses have shown to be successful (Nutma, 2019). Previously, doctors used standardized implants which they had to manually customize to fit the patient via bone grafting or using tools to mold the implant to fit the desired area (Ventola, 2014). 3D printing makes this process much simpler, as x-ray, MRI and CT scans can be translated into digital 3D printable designs (Ventola, 2014). This allows 3D printers to quickly generate customized implants and prostheses, thereby preventing the need for doctors to customize them manually. Dental, spinal and hip implants have been created using this method. Recently, 3D printed cranial implants have also been used, as each individual's unique skull shape makes it harder for surgeons to utilize standardized cranial implants (Ventola, 2014). Aside from these, 3D printing has also generated many other simple things used in the human body, such as a heart valve, spinal disk, an artificial ear, and a knee meniscus (Ventola, 2014). Evidently, 3D printing has many applications within the medical field beyond manufacturing PPE. As the technology improves and develops, its applications within the medical field will continue to grow.

# Chapter 15

## THE DRAWBACKS, LIMITATIONS, AND AREAS OF IMPROVEMENT OF 3D PRINTING TECHNOLOGY

As explained in the previous chapters, 3D printing is an incredibly versatile technology that holds enormous potential. With the PPE shortages spreading throughout the globe, 3D printing has demonstrated a variety of ways by which it is able to help alleviate the issue. However, as with all things, 3D printing has its own drawbacks that must be considered and concerns that must be addressed. This chapter will investigate the various disadvantages, concerns, limitations, and areas of improvement for 3D printing to provide a more detailed idea of what 3D printing truly entails as well as how it can be further optimized.

Beginning with the environmental implications of 3D printing, the full extent of the environmental impacts of additive manufacturing has yet to be investigated (Khosravani, 2020). Although it is believed that 3D printing is generally an efficient and sustainable technology, there are a variety of potentially hazardous and environmentally harmful consequences that need to be addressed (Liu et al., 2016). For instance, the energy consumption of 3D printing appears to be one of the largest concerns for manufacturers that are trying to improve the sustainability of this process (Khosravani, 2020). When compared to other manufacturing methods, such as injection molding, 3D printing tends to consume more electrical energy with large scale production (Khosravani, 2020). However, it is noteworthy that the amount of electrical energy required may vary due to a variety of factors, including the type of material used, the layer thickness, the speed of the printer, and many others (Khosravani, 2020). Regarding the type of material used, energy usage of a 3D printer can be influenced by the heat capacities of the materials (Khosravani, 2020). In essence, this property describes the energy required to change the temperature of a material by one degree (Hanrahan, 2012). Materials with low heat capacities would require less energy to heat up while materials with high heat capacities would require more energy. Therefore, one possible method to improve the energy efficiency of this technology is to make a larger effort to find and use materials that have low heat capacities. However, it is important to note that this is simply one possible approach and that there are many other solutions that could potentially be more effective, such as adding cooling channels to the structure of the product and reducing the weight of the printed part. Thus, further research is required to find new solutions relating to the various other factors that contribute to the energy consumption of 3D printing.

Moreover, another major concern involving the environmental implications of 3D printing is the potential emission of harmful chemicals, such as volatile organic compounds (VOCs) and nanoparticles (Khosravani, 2020). As previously mentioned in the earlier chapters, fused deposition modeling (FDM) is one of the many techniques of additive manufacturing and it is currently the most affordable and widely used method for 3D printing (Khosravani, 2020; Palermo, 2013b). In essence, this technique involves the melting of a thermoplastic, where it is fed into a high temperature nozzle (Khosravani, 2020). Afterwards, the molten material is then deposited onto the build platform to form the desired product (Palermo, 2013b). During this extrusion process, the thermal degradation of polymers and additives result in VOC emission (Khosravani, 2020). This presents an issue for those that own 3D printers as certain VOCs can cause harm to human health. One such VOC is styrene, which is emitted from the thermal processing of acrylonitrile butadiene styrene (ABS) high-impact polystyrene (HIPS) filaments (Azimi et al., 2016). With ABS being one of the most popular 3D printing materials in the world, those who operate 3D printers need to be extra cautious, as a study published in the Environmental Science & Technology Journal had found that styrene was among the top three VOCs that had been emitted in the largest quantities, reporting an emission rate that ranges from roughly 10 to 110 µg/min (Azimi et al., 2016). According to the study, the "worst-case scenario" with the largest styrene emission rate would result in a predicted styrene concentration that is "more than 20 times higher than the average concentration in U.S. residences". This presents an issue as the National Institute of Health (NIH) has reported that short-term exposure to styrene can result in negative respiratory effects, gastrointestinal effects, and cause irritation of the eyes, nose and skin (NIH, 2017). Long-term exposure, on the other hand, can lead to central nervous system and kidney damage, headaches, depression, and hearing loss, among many others (NIH, 2017). With styrene also being classified as a potential human carcinogen by the International Agency for Research on Cancer, it is clear that special precautions need to be taken to limit the exposure to these harmful VOCs (Azimi et al., 2016).

One possible solution to overcome this problem is to use nontoxic thermoplastic materials, such as biopolymer filaments (Khosravani, 2020). These materials are also a more environmentally friendly option as they are biodegradable and they can require a lower printing temperature, thereby reducing the overall energy consumption of the 3D printer (Khosravani, 2020). Additionally, biopolymer filaments can also be produced locally and offer financial advantages by reducing shipping costs (Khosravani, 2020). However, the current selection of biopolymer filaments available for 3D printing is quite limited which is why further research is needed to improve the safety and sustainability of 3D printing (Khosravani, 2020). Until then, other possible solutions that people can take to limit their exposure to VOCs is to improve the ventilation of 3D printing workspaces, utilize gas and particle filtration systems, and wear PPE when operating 3D printers (Azimi et al., 2016; Khosravani, 2020). Since the majority of commercially available desktop 3D printers utilize FDM technology, the fact they are currently being used in offices, homes, and classrooms, demonstrates that there is a significant health concern (Azimi et al., 2016; Khosravani, 2020). For this reason, rules and regulations need to be put into place to ensure that people are well protected from harmful chemicals and further research needs to be conducted to investigate the full extent of the toxicity and effects of these emissions.

Additionally, the sterilization of 3D printed PPE is another major concern as contaminated or insufficiently sterilized PPE can pose a large health risk to both patients and medical professionals. Part of this concern may stem from the difficulty in sterilizing porous materials (Tarfaoui et al., 2020). Since the extrusion process of FDM can cause the 3D printed material to be porous in nature, the subsequent internal geometry of the PPE may be very complex (Tarfaoui et al., 2020). With an increased surface area and an extensive network of tortuous pathways, sterilization becomes a much more difficult task (Tarfaoui et al., 2020). Consequently, microbes may be able to linger in the internal structure of the 3D printed PPE which could potentially lead to serious health issues (Tarfaoui et al., 2020). For this reason, it is crucial that adequate sterilization measures are taken to avoid causing further harm to others. However, there is also a large challenge in determining the precise method of sterilization that should be used for 3D printed PPE. This is because both the materials and the method of 3D printing used can influence the selection of sterilization approaches. For instance, thermal sterilization is often avoided for PPE that were manufactured through FDM technology as thermoplastics with low melting points are commonly used during this type of production (Skrzypczak et al., 2020; Tino et al., 2020). By exposing this material to high temperatures, the plastic would be vulnerable to deformations. Although there are high temperature 3D printers that can manufacture heat-resistant PPE, these printers have high costs which make them generally inaccessible to the average person (Skrzypczak et al., 2020). For this reason, alternative methods, such as the use of chemical disinfectants, ionizing radiation and hydrogen peroxide gas plasma, are much more preferred whenever these sterilization approaches are possible (Skrzypczak et al., 2020; Tino et al., 2020). However, due to the significant uncertainty regarding the efficacy of sterilization protocols for 3D printed PPEs, further research needs to be conducted to ensure that these PPEs are not doing more harm than good (Clifton et al., 2020; Skrzypczak et al., 2020).

Furthermore, another area of concern regarding 3D printed PPEs involves its effectiveness at preventing the spread of diseases. According to a recent official statement by the Food and Drug Administration, "3D-printed PPE are unlikely to provide the same fluid barrier and air filtration protection as FDA-cleared surgical masks and N95 respirators" (Clifton et al., 2020). Although there are downloadable PPE designs that have been reviewed for clinical use, there are also a number of other designs that can be found throughout the internet that lack validation and testing (Clifton et al., 2020; Manero et al., 2020). This presents a large issue as without a proper review of these designs, the efficacy of these 3D printed PPEs will remain uncertain. Therefore, those that wear these PPEs may be at risk of contracting or spreading the disease due to the possibility of inadequate protection. Moreover, there are also important aspects of traditional PPE that cannot be easily replicated through 3D printing. For instance, the filter media used in masks may be electrostatically charged to trap small particles that may attempt to travel through the filter (Gallagher, 2020). Since viruses and bacteria can use these small particles as a means to travel, the filter media can effectively block them, thus preventing the spread of diseases (Gallagher, 2020). Unfortunately, these electrostatic properties are difficult to reproduce through 3D printing and as stated by Health Canada, these 3D printed masks are "unlikely to provide the same fluid barrier and air filtration protection as licensed surgical masks or N95 respirators" (Clifton et al., 2020; Health Canada, 2020c). Although 3D printed masks are still capable of providing a physical barrier and offer some protection to the user, the extent of this protection remains debatable (Health Canada, 2020c). Evidently, the concerns surrounding 3D printed PPE are not unwarranted and further research is required to confirm the efficacy of various online designs as well as to improve the reproducibility of the key aspects of traditional PPE.

Lastly, the final concern that this chapter will investigate relates to the government's attitude towards 3D printed PPEs and the kinds of government regulations that have been put into place to ensure safety and effectiveness. With various news reports of PPE being 3D printed by non-traditional PPE manufacturers, such as volunteer organizations and academic institutions, there have been considerable concerns regarding whether or not these producers are meeting the health and safety standards that have been set out by the government (Thompson, 2020). In response, Health Canada (2020c) has clarified to the public that they are committed to regulating this process as they have stated:

> While Health Canada supports efforts to increase the availability of PPEs for frontline health workers, organizations should be aware that the manufacture of medical devices sold in Canada have technical considerations to ensure that they are safe, effective and of high quality and must meet certain regulatory standards.

Following this statement, Health Canada attempts to address the concerns by explaining how exactly this process is regulated. As described by Health Canada, there are two pathways by which a manufacturer can gain authorization to manufacture Class I medical devices, which includes the majority of PPEs. The manufacturer must either hold a Medical Establishment Device License (MDEL) or have authorization under the Interim Order (IO) respecting the importation and sale of medical devices for use in relation to COVID-19 (Health Canada, 2020c). Essentially, the difference between the two pathways is that the IO has fewer requirements than MDEL as it was designed to expedite the application process (Mensley, 2020; Tétrault, 2020). Despite this difference, however, Health Canada (2020c) assures the public that the PPE will comply with the standards as both pathways require product testing by a laboratory or certification body that has been accredited by the Standards Council of Canada. Additionally, Health Canada also clarifies that even under "urgent manufacturing scenarios", there are minimum specifications that manufacturers are expected to adhere to. However, it is important to note that since the word of choice was "expected", it is unclear if this would be heavily enforced or enforced at all. Seemingly, while there are valid concerns regarding the safety and effectiveness of 3D printed PPE, there has been a considerable effort made by the government to regulate this process and ensure that the frontline workers are provided with PPE that are safe to use and up to standard.

In conclusion, it is evident that 3D printing is not a perfect solution to the PPE crisis. From its environmental implications to the concerns regarding its effectiveness and sterilization, there are various drawbacks and limitations associated with the use of this technology. However, with the widespread use of 3D printing as a means to reduce this large deficit of PPE, it appears as though many people believe that the benefits of this technology outweigh the cons. With the potential to save lives and provide frontline workers with the protection that they desperately need, this mindset is not difficult to understand. However, this should not diminish the fact that there are still several drawbacks that must be addressed. Although 3D printing may never be the perfect solution to this crisis, by acknowledging the issues and actively seeking ways to improve this technology, 3D printing may become far more effective than what was initially believed possible.

# Chapter 16

## CONCLUSION

With the first couple chapters highlighting the large sacrifices being made by healthcare providers, it is understandable that there are many people in local communities that want to demonstrate their gratitude. This is especially evident in the case of the widespread PPE shortages as eager volunteers throughout the world have dedicated their time, effort, and resources to supply frontline workers with this desperately needed protection. One way by which they have attempted to achieve this is by harnessing the technology of additive manufacturing. Due to the shortage of masks, many health care providers are forced to re-use their masks for a long time. With 3D printing having a much quicker set-up time, as compared to other manufacturing methods, it has been able to rapidly begin manufacturing PPE to help meet the large immediate demand. Consequently, this has led many people to believe that 3D printing is the solution to the PPE crisis and that more investments should be made in this technology. However, with a claim being as bold as to say that 3D printing is the solution to the crisis, it is important to explore the implications of this technology.

In the earlier chapters, the book had attempted to provide the context behind the PPE shortage and the COVID-19 pandemic. Beginning with a general overview of the pandemic, the chapter explored a variety of topics, ranging from its recent history to the public health measures that the government have implemented to limit the spread of the virus. With this context of the social, economic, and health implications of the COVID-19 pandemic, the subsequent chapter had then transitioned to the varying responses and situations throughout the world. Since different countries have different political systems, manufacturing capabilities, economic power and values, it is not difficult to understand that the response to the PPE crisis may vary throughout the world. For this reason, this chapter had explored the four most affected countries, in terms of the number of confirmed COVID-19 cases, to highlight common themes and differences throughout the world. Afterwards, the book had then pivoted to the importance of preventative measures and the research behind them. Although these measures were implemented to limit the spread of the virus and to protect the wellbeing of its citizens, many have protested the new rules as an infringement of their constitutional rights to not follow the measures put in place. Regardless of the belief, however, the importance of preventative measures remains the same as limiting the number of COVID-19 cases is crucial in preventing a complete collapse of an already PPE-depleted healthcare system. Thus, it is not only important to supply frontline workers with the desperately needed PPEs, but to also limit the spread of this pandemic to prevent a further rise in the demand for PPE.

The next portion of the book focuses on the history and the different methods of 3D printing, which is crucial to understand as it is necessary for the reader to have a rudimentary understanding of what 3D printing truly entails before examining its specific use with regards to the PPE shortage. For this reason, this section begins by providing a brief overview of the development of the 3D printing technology and its growing applications in the medical field. With an understanding of how 3D printing has evolved through the years, the book then pivots its focus to the different methods of 3D printing. Although 3D printing is commonly referred to as a single technology, there are various methods with different advantages and disadvantages. Beginning with the methods of SLA, FDM, and SLS, this chapter examines these different techniques to provide a basic understanding of what they are as well as which method may be the most appropriate choice for the ongoing PPE crisis. Next, the following chapter then discusses another method of 3D printing, known as Polymer Jet Fabrication. This technique is capable of manufacturing a large variety of products, ranging from PPEs to vaccines and medication.

After this basic introduction to the field of 3D printing, the book then transitions to explore various other manufacturing techniques which could be used as either an alternative to 3D printing or as a technology that can be optimized through

3D printing. This section of the book focuses on the following methods: Injection molding, stamping, and hydroforming. In the injection molding chapter, it was made clear that the substantially lower setup time and costs of 3D printing was a significant advantage. However, in the long run, injection molding would be a far more advantageous manufacturing approach as it is much more cost effective with large scale production. Thus, the chapter had concluded that the rapid response of 3D printing should be used during the early stages of the PPE shortage to optimize injection molding processes and to meet the large immediate demand of PPE. With this approach, the manufacturers would have enough time to increase their injection molding capabilities and produce a sufficient volume of PPE. In the case of stamping and hydroforming, on the other hand, these manufacturing techniques are not nearly as important in the context of the PPE shortages as they are rarely used to produce PPE. While there is a possibility of producing PPE through stamping techniques, in the case of hydroforming, it is quite rare as metal is the predominant material used for this manufacturing method. However, that is not to say that they do not play a role in COVID-19 pandemic as they can be used to manufacture other types of equipment that are crucial in healthcare facilities.

With an introductory understanding of the various manufacturing techniques and the relationship that they may have with 3D printing technology, the book then shifts its focus to the different types of PPE. Starting with the topic of face masks, this section explored the importance of cloth and surgical masks and compared the 3D printing process to the regular manufacturing of masks. This was done in terms of cost, production duration, and efficiency. Afterwards, the following chapter had then explored the topic of N95 respirators. Since N95 respirators are more effective than both surgical and cloth masks, due to their filtration process, N95 respirators are critically important for frontline workers. However, with the import of N95 masks being threatened by the US government, the application of 3D printing technology has been investigated so that countries can be more self-reliant and ensure that they have a steady supply of these crucially important PPEs. Additionally, the chapter also explores the use of face shields and masks with visors. With many healthcare professionals being forced to wear the same mask for extended periods of time, the physical protection offered by face shields and visors can help extend the lifespan of the mask. With this type of PPE being reusable, disposable, easily manufactured, and fairly inexpensive, the use of face shields and masks with visors have significantly grown in popularity with the spread of the COVID-19 pandemic. Lastly, the final types of PPEs discussed in this section are hazmat suits and gloves.

Since both of these PPEs protect against more significant biohazards, manufacturers must meet a high level of standard in order to distribute their products. For this reason, 3D printing technology is not currently being used to manufacture hazmat suits and gloves as this technology has yet to mature to such advanced levels. However, with time and further developments in the field, it is possible for hazmat suits and gloves to be 3D printed in the near future.

Finally, with a basic understanding of the various types of PPEs, the last section of the book discussed how 3D printing can be used to further improve the effectiveness of the equipment as well as examine the concerns and limitations surrounding the use of this technology with regards to 3D printing PPE. As previously mentioned, one of the many benefits of 3D printing is its seemingly limitless freedom of manufacturing complex shapes. With this ability, PPE can be customized for different people in different ways and for different settings. This is a significant advantage as PPEs, such as masks, can be specifically designed to fit the exact parameters of an individual's face to offer more effective protection. With all these advantages making 3D printing seem as though it is the perfect solution, the final chapter focuses specifically on the concerns and limitations of this technology to provide the reader with a more comprehensive understanding of what the use of this technology truly entails. By the end of the chapter, it is clear that there are numerous potential issues with using 3D printing as a means to manufacture PPE. However, with the lives of thousands of frontline workers being at risk due to an insufficient supply of PPE, many would consider the benefits to outweigh the cons. Regardless of whether or not this may be true, further research should still be conducted to address those concerns and make 3D printing a much more effective technology. Although this book had predominantly focused on the applications of 3D printing in the medical field, it is also important to recognize its advancements in other disciplines. In education, 3D printing has been implemented in many school curriculums as it allows students to further enhance their creative skills by making inexpensive prototypes (MakerBot, 2019). The use of 3D printers in the classroom nurtures the need for more hands-on experiences and bridges the gap between picture and reality. Additionally, with the use of this technology becoming more common in the classroom, students can gain greater exposure to the field of STEM and strengthen their interest (MakerBot, 2019).

In addition to the field of education, this technology is also commonly used in prototyping and manufacturing (MakerBot, 2019). As previously discussed, manufacturing technology often requires a prototype or a model during the planning stages of a project. Since 3D printing is remarkably more cost effective than traditional manufacturing processes, with regards to small scale production, additive manufacturing would be a more ideal approach for developing prototypes. Moreover, the freedom that 3D printing offers by producing objects from digital designs is another significant benefit as it allows for adjustments and improvements to be easily made. Additionally, another field where the use of 3D printing has grown in popularity is the construction field (MakerBot, 2019). In 2017, the first residential building that was fully constructed using a 3D printer had occurred in Yaroslavl, Russia (MakerBot, 2019). The parts of the building were individually 3D printed and assembled at the construction site. With such a monumental application of 3D printing technology, it is clear that the future of additive manufacturing is truly limitless, and that 3D printing will play an increasingly important role in all aspects of society.

As it has been described throughout the book, 3D printing is a powerful technology that has been used to address the PPE shortage. While it is clear that this technology has demonstrated significant improvement through the years, there are also several other examples of technological advances and research that have helped us be better prepared for the COVID-19 pandemic. For instance, during the SARS (Severe Acute Respiratory Syndrome) epidemic, which began in 2002 and lasted until the year 2004, there was a long period of time between the beginning of the outbreak and the development diagnostic tests (Dutton, 2020). Interestingly, out of the three attempts made, two of the diagnostic test attempts could only be used in the later course of disease and one was outright unsuccessful (Dutton, 2020). In comparison, the diagnostic tests for COVID-19 were able to be developed and used within a few months as researchers had transferred their knowledge from the SARS epidemic. (Dutton, 2020). With such a vast improvement between the two instances, it is reasonable to assume that through the lessons and knowledge learned from this pandemic, governments and public health systems will be much more prepared to handle the inevitable future outbreak of a novel disease.

With a COVID-19 vaccine being far from sight, the rapid spread of this disease has caused many people to be overwhelmed with feelings of panic and helplessness. As the situation worsened, the medical community was under immense pressure to help save and treat the unfortunate members of their communities. However, as the number of COVID-19 cases increased, the demand for PPEs soared, resulting in a large international shortage. To help combat this crisis, several volunteers and organizations have stepped in, many of which have utilized the power of 3D printing. Although 3D printing has many drawbacks and is far from being the perfect solution, its ability to provide a swift response is seemingly unparalleled by any other manufacturing method. With further improvements and research in this field, one can only imagine what the future of 3D printing may hold.

# References

3D Insider. (n.d.). The 9 Different Types of 3D Printers. https://3dinsider.com/3d-printer-types/

Adelman, S., Bapat, A., Bertisch, S., Bojarski, E., Ellerin, T., Farid, H., Gabbay, R., Glazer, E. S., Grinspoon, P., Katz-Wise, S. L., Komaroff, A., Krakower, D., LaPlante, D., LeWine, H. E., Lewis, D. K. L., Liu, K., Marcus, J., Marques, L., McCarthy, C., … Wolfson, A. R. (2020). Coronavirus Resource Center. Harvard Health Publishing. https://www.health.harvard.edu/diseases-and-conditions/coronavirus-resource-center

Ahart, M. (2019, June 3). Types of 3D Printing Explained. Proto Labs. https://www.protolabs.com/resources/blog/types-of-3d-printing/

Ahmetoglu, M. (2001, March 5). The basic elements of tubular hydroforming. The Fabricator. https://www.thefabricator.com/thefabricator/article/hydroforming/the-basic-elements-of-tubular-hydroforming

Alongi, P. (2014, December 16). Clemson University's 'bioprinting' central to new businesses. Clemson University. https://newsstand.clemson.edu/clemson-universitys-bioprinting-central-to-new-businesses/

Alspach, K. (2020, March 26). HP CEO Enrique Lores Sees Permanent Changes, 'Significant Tailwind' From Coronavirus Crisis. CRN. https://www.crn.com/news/mobility/hp-ceo-enrique-lores-sees-permanent-changes-significant-tailwind-from-coronavirus-crisis.

Alverez, P., Devine, C., Griffin, D., & Holmes, K. (2020, July 14). Trump administration's delayed use of 1950s law leads to critical supplies shortages. CNN. https://www.cnn.com/2020/07/13/politics/delayed-use-defense-production-act-ppe-shortages/index.html

American Hydroformers. (n.d.). What is Hydroforming. https://americanhydroformers.com/what-is-hydroforming/

American Hydroformers. (2014, January 30). 7 Benefits of Hydroforming. https://americanhydroformers.com/benefits-of-hydroforming/

Arrowsmith, R. (2014, June 10). Injection Molding: A Mainstay. Medical Product Outsourcing. https://www.mpo-mag.com/issues/2014-06-01/view_features/injection-molding-a-mainstay/

Azimi, P., Zhao, D., Pouzet, C., Crain, N. E., & Stephens, B. (2016). Emissions of Ultrafine Particles and Volatile Organic Compounds from Commercially Available Desktop Three-Dimensional Printers with Multiple Filaments. Environmental Science & Technology, 50(3), 1260–1268. https://doi.org/10.1021/acs.est.5b04983

Barrow Neurological Institution. (n.d.). 3D Printed N95 Replacement Mask. https://www.barrowneuro.org/get-to-know-barrow/barrow-innovation-center-2/3d-printed-n95-mask/

BBC. (2020, April 3). Coronavirus: US 'wants 3M to end mask exports to Canada and Latin America'. https://www.bbc.com/news/world-us-canada-52161032

BBC. (2020, July 20). Customised 3D printed masks: A more comfortable fit? https://www.bbc.com/news/av/technology-53432848

Benitez-Rangel, J. P., Domínguez-González, A., Herrera-Ruiz, G., & Delgado-Rosas, M. (2007). Filling Process in Injection Mold: A Review. Polymer-Plastics Technology and Engineering, 46(7), 721–727. https://doi.org/10.1080/15583720701271641

Bennett, M. (2018, October 15). The Healthy State of the Plastics Industry. JPMorgan Chase & Co. https://www.jpmorgan.com/commercial-banking/insights/plastics-industry-vol17

Bensadoun, E. (2020, April 1). Coronavirus: Can Canada get front-line health workers what they need before it's too late? Global News. https://globalnews.ca/news/6745915/coronavirus-personal-protective-equipment-needs/

Berman, B. (2012). 3-D printing: The new industrial revolution. Business Horizons, 55(2), 155–162. https://doi.org/10.1016/j.bushor.2011.11.003

Birks, S. (2014, November 3). Opinion: What is the real cost of a hazmat suit? Cleanroom Technology. https://www.cleanroomtechnology.com/news/article_page/Opinion_What_is_the_real_cost_of_a_hazmat_suit/103067#:~:text=The%20cost%20of%20a%20full,CERPs)%20and%20the%20expenses%20mount

Boissonneault, T. (2020, March 25). Canadian government calls for help for COVID-19 supplies. 3D Printing Media Network. https://www.3dprintingmedia.network/canadian-government-covid-19-supplies-help/

Boynton, S. (2020, July 23). As U.S. hits 4 million coronavirus cases in record time, deaths are also surging. Global News. https://globalnews.ca/news/7212352/us-coronavirus-4-million-cases/

Bozard, J. (n.d.). Stamping or 3D Printing? Phoenix Specialty. https://www.phoenixspecialty.com/resources/blog/stamping-or-3d-printing

Brezinová, J., & Guzanová, A. (2010). Friction Conditions during the Wear of Injection Mold Functional Parts in Contact with Polymer Composites. Journal of Reinforced Plastics and Composites, 29(11), 1712–1726. https://doi.org/10.1177/0731684409341675

Center of Disease Control and Prevention (CDC). (n.d.). Developmental Milestones https://www.cdc.gov/ncbddd/childdevelopment/positiveparenting/infants.html

Center of Disease Control and Prevention (CDC). (2004, January 13). SARS Basics Factsheet. https://www.cdc.gov/sars/about/fs-sars.html

Center of Disease Control and Prevention (CDC). (2020a). Symptoms of Coronavirus. https://www.cdc.gov/coronavirus/2019-ncov/symptoms-testing/symptoms.html

Center of Disease Control and Prevention (CDC). (2020b). When to Wear Gloves. https://www.cdc.gov/coronavirus/2019-ncov/prevent-getting-sick/gloves.html

Center of Disease Control and Prevention (CDC). (2020c, August 14). People with Certain Medical Conditions. https://www.cdc.gov/coronavirus/2019-ncov/need-extra-precautions/people-with-medical-conditions.html

Chen, Y. (2020, March 21). 3D Printed Injection Mold: All You Need to Know. All3DP. https://all3dp.com/2/3d-printed-injection-mold/

Chen, Z., & Turng, L.-S. (2005). A review of current developments in process and quality control for injection molding. Advances in Polymer Technology, 24(3), 165–182. https://doi.org/10.1002/adv.20046

Christian, J. (2020, March 15). WE ASKED EXPERTS WHETHER YOU SHOULD WEAR A HAZMAT SUIT IN PUBLIC. Futurism. https://futurism.com/neoscope/grocery-stores-hazmat-suits

Clifton, W., Damon, A., & Martin, A. K. (2020). Considerations and Cautions for Three-Dimensional-Printed Personal Protective Equipment in the COVID-19 Crisis. 3D Printing and Additive Manufacturing, 7(3), 97–99. https://doi.org/10.1089/3dp.2020.0101

Copper 3D. (n.d.). Hack The Pandemic. https://copper3d.com/hackthepandemic/

CustomPartNet. (n.d.). Injection Molding. https://www.custompartnet.com/wu/InjectionMolding

Dawkins, D. (2020, June 10). Diesel Spill Could Cost Billionaire Potanin $4 Billion - Russia's Richest Man To 'Clean Up' His Own Mess. Forbes. https://www.forbes.com/sites/daviddawkins/2020/06/10/billionaire-vladimir-potanin-promises-to-clean-up-his-mess--diesel-fuel-spill-could-cost-russias-richest-man-4-billion/#50d937ba6f14

DeClerq, K. (2020, June 30). What you need to know about Toronto's mandatory mask policy. CTV News. https://toronto.ctvnews.ca/what-you-need-to-know-about-toronto-s-mandatory-mask-policy-1.5006032

Diaz, D., Sands, G. & Alesci, C. (2020, April 16). Protective equipment costs increase over 1,000% amid competition and surge in demand. CNN. https://www.cnn.com/2020/04/16/politics/ppe-price-costs-rising-economy-personal-protective-equipment/index.html

Dunn, L. & Fitzpatrick, S. (2020, June 12). Few N95 masks, reused gowns: Dire PPE shortages reveal COVID-

19's racial divide. NBC News.

https://www.nbcnews.com/health/health-care/few-n95-masks-reused-gowns-dire-ppe-shortages-reveal-covid-n1229546

DuPont (n.d.). DuPont⬜ Tychem® garments for lightweight protection from chemical and biological hazards. https://www.dupont.co.uk/personal-protection/tychem.html

DuPont Tyvek (n.d.). What is Tyvek®. https://www.dupont.com/tyvekdesign/design-with-tyvek/why-tyvek.html

Dutton, G. (2020, April 3). Compare: 2003 SARS Pandemic Versus 2020 COVID-19 Pandemic. BioSpace. https://www.biospace.com/article/comparison-2003-sars-pandemic-vs-2020-covid-19-pandemic/

Dwyer, D. & Yoo, J. (2020, April 9). Making 'PPE' at home: Families use 3D printers to address coronavirus shortages. ABC News. https://abcnews.go.com/Politics/making-ppe-home-families-3d-printers-address-coronavirus/story?id=69995774

Dyer, O. (2020). Covid-19: Cases rise in Russia as health workers pay the price for PPE shortage. BMJ, 369. https://doi.org/10.1136/bmj.m1975

Eagle Protect. (2018, December 12). The True Cost of a Disposable Glove. https://blog.eagleprotect.com/the-true-cost-of-a-disposable-glove

Elliott, J. K. (2020, May 21). Nurse with swimsuit under her clear gown exposes coronavirus PPE issues in Russia. Global News. https://globalnews.ca/news/6968452/coronavirus-nurse-russia-hot-ppe/

Engineering Specialities, Inc. (ESI). (n.d.). What Is Metal Stamping? https://www.esict.com/what-is-metal-stamping/

Evans, P. (2020, March 27). How bad will Canada's Recession be? CBC. https://www.cbc.ca/news/business/covid-19-recession-economy-analysis-1.5510596

Fagundes, M. (2020, May 21). Covid-19 Is Killing Nurses in Brazil More Than Anywhere Else. Bloomberg. https://www.bloomberg.com/news/articles/2020-05-21/covid-19-is-killing-nurses-in-brazil-more-than-anywhere-else

Farmer, B. & Wallen J. (2020, April 9). Doctors in India and Pakistan wear bin bags and raincoats to protect against Covid-19. The Telegraph. https://www.telegraph.co.uk/global-health/science-and-disease/doctors-india-pakistan-wear-bin-bags-raincoats-protect-against/

Farr, C. (2020, July 22). Brazil turned the coronavirus into a political football, with devastating results. CNBC. https://www.cnbc.com/2020/07/22/brazil-politics-mixed-messages-hurt-response.html

Fonseca, P. & Paraguassu, L. (2020, May 12). Brazil's coronavirus cases pass Germany's as Bolsonaro fights to open gyms. Reuters. https://www.reuters.com/article/us-health-coronavirus-brazil/brazils-coronavirus-cases-pass-germanys-as-bolsonaro-fights-to-open-gyms-idUSKBN22O34J

France-Presse, A. (2020, May 4). Coronavirus: Brazil's Bolsonaro eggs on huge crowd of lockdown protesters, blames governors for 'destroying jobs'. South China Morning Post. https://www.scmp.com/news/world/americas/article/3082699/coronavirus-brazils-bolsonaro-eggs-huge-crowd-lockdown

Franchetti, M., & Kress, C. (2017). An economic analysis comparing the cost feasibility of replacing injection molding processes with emerging additive manufacturing techniques. The International Journal of Advanced Manufacturing Technology, 88(9), 2573–2579. https://doi.org/10.1007/s00170-016-8968-7

Fluid Forming Americas. (n.d.). HYDROFORMING FOR HEALTHCARE & MEDICAL EQUIPMENT INDUSTRY. https://www.ffamericas.com/medical-equipment/

Gitlin, J. M. (2020, June 18). GM makes cars; how did it quickly pivot to face shields and ventilators? Ars Technica. https://arstechnica.com/cars/2020/06/gm-makes-cars-how-did-it-quickly-pivot-to-face-shields-and-ventilators/

Gallagher, M. B. (2020, March 26). 3 Questions: The risks of using 3D printing to make personal protective equipment. Massachusetts Institute of Technology (MIT) News. http://news.mit.edu/2020/3q-risks-using-3d-printing-make-personal-protective-equipment-0326

Gan, W. H., Lim, J. W., & Koh, D. (2020). Preventing Intra-hospital Infection and Transmission of Coronavirus Disease 2019 in Health-care Workers. Safety and Health at Work, 11(2), 241–243. https://doi.org/10.1016/j.shaw.2020.03.001

GlobeNewswire (2018, July 18). Global Disposable Medical Gloves Market 2016-2024: Top Glove - The Largest Rubber Glove Manufacturer. https://www.globenewswire.com/news-release/2018/07/18/1538755/0/en/Global-Disposable-Medical-Gloves-Market-2016-2024-Top-Glove-The-Largest-Rubber-Glove-Manufacturer.html

GloveNation. (n.d.). Sterile vs. Non-Sterile Gloves. https://glovenation.com/blogs/default-blog/sterile-vs-non-sterile-gloves

Goldberg, D. (2018, April 13). History of 3D Printing: It's Older Than You Are (That Is, If You're Under 30). Autodesk. https://www.autodesk.com/redshift/history-of-3d-printing/

Government of Canada. (2020a). Coronavirus disease (COVID-19). https://www.canada.ca/en/public-health/services/diseases/coronavirus-disease-covid-19.html

Government of Canada. (2020b). Coronavirus disease (COVID-19): Prevention and risks. https://www.canada.ca/en/public-health/services/diseases/2019-novel-coronavirus-infection/prevention-risks.html#h

Government of Canada. (2020c). Coronavirus disease (COVID-19): Symptoms and treatment. https://www.canada.ca/en/public-health/services/diseases/2019-novel-coronavirus-infection/symptoms.html

Gray, R. (2020, August 6). Why a face shield alone may not protect you from coronavirus. BBC News. https://www.bbc.com/future/article/20200806-are-face-shields-effective-against-covid-19

Gregurić, L. (2019a, June 29). PolyJet – 3D Printing Technologies Simply Explained. All3DP. https://all3dp.com/2/polyjet-3d-printing-technologies-simply-explained/.

Gregurić, L. (2019b, October 5). History of 3D Printing: When Was 3D Printing Invented? All3DP. https://all3dp.com/2/history-of-3d-printing-when-was-3d-printing-invented/

Hanrahan, G. (2012). Aqueous Chemistry. In Key Concepts in Environmental Chemistry (pp. 73–106). Elsevier. https://doi.org/10.1016/B978-0-12-374993-2.10003-2

Hanson, K. (2019, October, 8). Plastic injection molds can be 3D-printed quickly. The Additive Report. https://www.thefabricator.com/additivereport/article/additive/plastic-injection-molds-can-be-3d-printed-quickly

Harm Reduction Coalition. (n.d.). Principles of Harm Reduction. https://harmreduction.org/about-us/principles-of-harm-reduction/

Health Canada. (2020a). Helping people who use substances during the COVID-19 pandemic. https://www.canada.ca/en/health-canada/services/substance-use/helping-people-who-use-substances-covid-19.html

Health Canada. (2020b). Personal protective equipment against COVID-19: Medical gloves. https://www.canada.ca/en/health-canada/services/drugs-health-products/covid19-industry/medical-devices/personal-protective-equipment/medical-gloves.html

Health Canada. (2020c, April 18). 3D printing and other manufacturing of personal protective equipment in response to COVID-19. https://www.canada.ca/en/health-canada/services/drugs-health-products/medical-devices/covid-19-unconventional-manufacturing-personal-protective-equipment.html

Hedrick, A. (2018, July 18). Die Basics 101: Intro to stamping. The Fabricator. https://www.thefabricator.com/thefabricator/article/stamping/die-basics-101-intro-to-stamping

Higgins-Dunn, N. & Kim, J. (2020, July 22). FEMA head says coronavirus hot spots may face PPE shortages, U.S. isn't 'out of the woods'. CNBC. https://www.cnbc.com/2020/07/22/fema-head-says-coronavirus-hotspots-may-face-ppe-shortages.html

Hyatt, J. S. & Hyatt, J. W. (1872). Improvement in Process and Apparatus for Manufacturing Pyroxyline (Patent 133 229). United States Patent Office.

Ishack, S. & Lipner, S. R. (2020, April 21). Applications of 3D Printing Technology to Address COVID-19–Related Supply Shortages. The American Journal of Medicine, 133(7), 771–773. https://doi.org/10.1016/j.amjmed.2020.04.002

Jacobs, A. (2020, July 8). Grave Shortages of Protective Gear Flare Again as Covid Cases Surge. The New York Times. https://www.nytimes.com/2020/07/08/health/coronavirus-masks-ppe-doc.html

Jahan, S. A., & El-Mounayri, H. (2016). Optimal Conformal Cooling Channels in 3D Printed Dies for Plastic Injection Molding. Procedia Manufacturing, 5, 888–900. https://doi.org/10.1016/j.promfg.2016.08.076

Jain, T. & Nair, A. S. (2020, April 24). DuPont doubles output of protective gowns to 30 million per month. Reuters. https://www.reuters.com/article/us-dupont-protective-gear/dupont-doubles-output-of-protective-gowns-to-30-million-per-month-idUSKCN22637F

James, C. (2020, April 4). ER doctor in New York details dire supply shortages from the front lines of the coronavirus fight. CNN. https://www.cnn.com/2020/03/31/us/coronavirus-medical-shortages-us/index.html

Johns Hopkins Center for Health Security. (2020, April 18). Assumptions. https://www.centerforhealthsecurity.org/resources/COVID-19/PPE/PPE-assumptions

Johns Hopkins Coronavirus Resource Center. (2020). COVID-19 Dashboard by the Center for Systems Science and Engineering (CSSE) at Johns Hopkins University (JHU). https://coronavirus.jhu.edu/map.html

Jones, A. M. (2020, July 28). WHO head says Canada has 'done well' at bringing COVID-19 under control. CTV News. https://www.ctvnews.ca/health/coronavirus/who-head-says-canada-has-done-well-at-bringing-covid-19-under-control-1.5042569

Jones Metal Products. (2015, December 14). 3D Printing and Additive Manufacturing for Hydroforming. https://www.jmpforming.com/blog/hydroforming/3d-printing-and-additive-manufacturing-for-hydroforming.htm

Jones Metal Products. (2017, July 28). Sheet Hydroforming vs. Tube Hydroforming Process. https://www.jmpforming.com/blog/hydroforming/sheet-hydroforming-vs-tube-hydroforming.htm

Kadakia, P. M. (2020, April 27). Covid-19 pushes 3D printing to new dimension. Forbes India. https://www.forbesindia.com/article/coronavirus/covid19-pushes-3d-printing-to-new-dimension/59039/1

Kale, S. (2020, March 26). 'They can cost £63k': how the hazmat suit came to represent disease, danger – and hope. The Guardian. https://www.theguardian.com/world/2020/mar/26/hazmat-suit-disease-deadly-viruses-danger-symbol-heroic

Kantis, C., Kiernan, S. & Bardi, J. S. (2020, July 27). UPDATED: Timeline of the Coronavirus. Think Global Health. https://www.thinkglobalhealth.org/article/updated-timeline-coronavirus

Khosravani, M. R., & Reinicke, T. (2020). On the environmental impacts of 3D printing technology. Applied Materials Today, 20, 100689. https://doi.org/10.1016/j.apmt.2020.100689

Khurshudyan, I. (2020, May 20). Two Russian doctors die after mysterious falls amid COVID-19 pressure, another critically hurt. National Post. https://nationalpost.com/health/two-russian-doctors-die-after-mysterious-falls-amid-covid-19-pressure-another-critically-hurt

Little, B. (2020, May 6). When Mask-Wearing Rules in the 1918 Pandemic Faced Resistance. History. https://www.history.com/news/1918-spanish-flu-mask-wearing-resistance.

Liu, Z., Jiang, Q., Zhang, Y., Li, T., & Zhang, H.-C. (2016, September 27). Sustainability of 3D Printing: A

Critical Review and Recommendations. ASME 2016 11th International Manufacturing Science and Engineering Conference. https://doi.org/10.1115/MSEC2016-8618

Lu, R., Zhao, X., Li, J., Niu, P., Yang, B., Wu, H., Wang, W., Song, H., Huang, B., Zhu, N., Bi, Y., Ma, X., Zhan, F., Wang, L., Hu, T., Zhou, H., Hu, Z., Zhou, W., Zhao, L., … Tan, W. (2020). Genomic characterisation and epidemiology of 2019 novel coronavirus: Implications for virus origins and receptor binding. The Lancet, 395(10224), 565–574. https://doi.org/10.1016/S0140-6736(20)30251-8

MakerBot. (2019, April 18). Top 3D Printing Applications Across Industries. https://www.makerbot.com/ stories/design/top-5-3d-printing-applications/

Manero, A., Smith, P., Koontz, A., Dombrowski, M., Sparkman, J., Courbin, D., & Chi, A. (2020). Leveraging 3D Printing Capacity in Times of Crisis: Recommendations for COVID-19 Distributed Manufacturing for Medical Equipment Rapid Response. International Journal of Environmental Research and Public Health, 17(13), 4634. https://doi.org/10.3390/ijerph17134634

Masood, S. (2014). Introduction to Advances in Additive Manufacturing and Tooling. Comprehensive Materials Processing, 10, 69-70. doi:10.1016/b978-0-08-096532-1.01016-5

Matisons, M. (2015, December 16). It's Easy to Make a 3D Printed Stamp, or Even a Whole Stamp Collection. 3DPrint.com. https://3dprint.com/110918/3d-printed-stamp-collection/

Mayo Clinic. (2020, June 06). Herd immunity and COVID-19 (coronavirus): What you need to know. https:// www.mayoclinic.org/diseases-conditions/coronavirus/in-depth/herd-immunity-and-coronavirus/art-20486808

McCarten, J. (2020, April 3). 3M says Trump officials have told it to stop sending face masks to Canada. Trudeau responds. National Post. https://nationalpost.com/news/world/3m-says-trump-officials-have-told-it-to-stop-sending-face-masks-to-canada

McGuigan, D. (2020, January 29). Plastic Injection Molding vs 3D Printing – Which is Better? Kaysun. https:// www.kaysun.com/blog/plastic-injection-molding-vs-3d-printing#:~:text=3D%20printing%20has%20 given%20engineers,runs%20of%20complex%20plastic%20designs

Mensley, M. (2020, April 9). Coronavirus Crisis: 3D Printing Community Responds. All3DP. https://all3dp. com/1/coronavirus-covid-19-sars-cov-2-3d-printing/

Milford, M. (2014, October 15). Market loves hazmat-suit makers after more Ebola in U.S. USA TODAY. https://www.usatoday.com/story/money/business/2014/10/15/ebola-protective-gear/17307415/

Mills, G. (n.d.). Understanding Metal Stamping. Thomas Industry. https://www.thomasnet.com/articles/ custom-manufacturing-fabricating/understanding-metal-stamping/

Mody, S. & Manning, P. (2020, February 21). DuPont ramps up safety suit production as coronavirus causes shortages in China. CNBC. https://www.cnbc.com/2020/02/21/coronavirus-dupont-ramps-up-safety-suit-production-amid-china-shortage.html

Moon, M. (2020, February 17). What you need to know about 3D-printed organs. Engadget. https://www. engadget.com/2014-06-20-3d-printed-organ-explainer.html

Moulson, G. (2020, June 14). Europe reopens many borders but not to Americans, Asians. CTV News. https:// www.ctvnews.ca/world/europe-reopens-many-borders-but-not-to-americans-asians-1.4983606

Mulvihill, G. & Fassett, C. (2020, July 8). Coronavirus: U.S. sees new shortage of PPE as cases, hospitalizations climb. Global News. https://globalnews.ca/news/7151297/coronavirus-us-ppe-shortage/

Mundell E. J. (2020, April 30). Should Face Shields Replace Face Masks to Ward Off Coronavirus? WebMD. https://www.webmd.com/lung/news/20200430/face-shields-a-more-effective-deterrent-to-covid#1

National Institute of Health (NIH). (2017, May 31). Styrene. https://toxtown.nlm.nih.gov/chemicals-and-contaminants/styrene

Nawrat, A. (2020, January 23). 3D printing in the medical field: Four major applications revolutionising the industry. Verdict Media. https://www.medicaldevice-network.com/features/3d-printing-in-the-medical-field-applications/

Novak, J. (2020, May 4). Millions of products have been 3D printed for the coronavirus pandemic – but they bring risks. The Conversation. https://theconversation.com/millions-of-products-have-been-3d-printed-for-the-coronavirus-pandemic-but-they-bring-risks-137486

Nutma, M. (2019, August 7). Why 3D printing is perfect for medical applications. HealthTechZone. https:// www.healthtechzone.com/topics/healthcare/articles/2019/08/07/442906-why-3d-printing-perfect-medical-applications.htm

O'Kane, C. (2020, March 20). Doctor who moved into his garage to protect newborn and family receives praise from Obama. CBS News. https://www.cbsnews.com/news/coronavirus-doctor-moved-into-garage-protect-newborn-family-president-barack-obama-praises-health-care-workers/

Pacific Metal Stampings. (n.d.). Metal Stampings for the Medical Industry. https://www.pacificmetalstampings. com/medical.html

Palermo, E. (2013a, August 13). What is Selective Laser Sintering? Live Science. https://www.livescience. com/38862-selective-laser-sintering.html

Palermo, E. (2013b, September 19). Fused Deposition Modeling: Most Common 3D Printing Method. Live Science. https://www.livescience.com/39810-fused-deposition-modeling.html

Pandey, V. (2020, April 13). Coronavirus: India's race against time to save doctors. BBC News. https://www.bbc. com/news/world-asia-india-52215071

Pearson, M. (2020, April 17). Stepping up during COVID-19: McMaster students step up to provide PPE for front-line health workers. The Hamilton Spectator. https://www.thespec.com/news/hamilton-region/2020/04/17/mcmaster-u-of-t-medical-students-step-up-to-provide-ppe-for-front-line-health-workers.html

Peek, K. (2020, June 2). How to Use Masks during the Coronavirus Pandemic. Scientific American. https://www.scientificamerican.com/article/how-to-use-masks-during-the-coronavirus-pandemic/.

Peel, M., McMorrow, R., Liu, N., Chazan, G., Mallet, V., Schipani, A., & Politi, J. (2020, April 7). EU warns of global bidding war for medical equipment. Financial Times. https://www.ft.com/content/a94aa917-f5a0-4980-a51a-28576f09410a

Petch, M. (2020, April 29). 3D Printing Community Responds to COVID-19 and Coronavirus Resources. 3D Printing Industry. https://3dprintingindustry.com/news/3d-printing-community-responds-to-covid-19-and-coronavirus-resources-169143/.

Petersen, E., Koopmans, M., Go, U., Hamer, D. H., Petrosillo, N., Castelli, F., Storgaard, M., Khalili, S. A., & Simonsen, L. (2020). Comparing SARS-CoV-2 with SARS-CoV and influenza pandemics. The Lancet Infectious Diseases, 0(0). https://doi.org/10.1016/S1473-3099(20)30484-9

Polyplastics (n.d.). The Outline of Injection Molding. https://www.polyplastics.com/en/support/mold/outline/index.html

Pomager, J. (2015, February 2). 3D-Printed Injection Molding: The Future Of Rapid Prototyping? Med Device Online. https://www.meddeviceonline.com/doc/3d-printed-injection-molding-the-future-of-rapid-prototyping-0001

Porterfield, C. (2020, April 29). A Lot Of PPE Doesn't Fit Women—And In The Coronavirus Pandemic, It Puts Them In Danger. Forbes. https://www.forbes.com/sites/carlieporterfield/2020/04/29/a-lot-of-ppe-doesnt-fit-women-and-in-the-coronavirus-pandemic-it-puts-them-in-danger/#773879e315a0

Proto3000. (n.d.). 3Technical Application Guide FDM Tooling for Sheet Metal Forming. https://proto3000.com/applications/3d-printing-guides-metal-forming-with-3d-printing/

Proto3000. (2020, March 12). PolyJet 3D Printing Technology. https://proto3000.com/service/3d-printing-services/technologies/polyjet/.

Public Health Ontario. (2020, July 16). COVID-19 Routes of Transmission – What We Know So Far. https://www.publichealthontario.ca/-/media/documents/ncov/wwksf-routes-transmission-mar-06-2020.pdf?la=en

Qian, Y., Willeke, K., Grinshpun, S. A., Donnelly, J., & Coffey, C. C. (1998). Performance of N95 Respirators: Filtration Efficiency for Airborne Microbial and Inert Particles. American Industrial Hygiene Association Journal, 59(2), 128–132. https://doi.org/10.1080/15428119891010389

Rainsford, S. (2020, April 28). Coronavirus: Putin admits PPE shortage as lockdown extended. BBC News. https://www.bbc.com/news/world-europe-52461431

Rathi, C. (2018, January 12). Traditional Manufacturing Vs 3d Printing. Precious 3D. https://precious3d.com/

traditional-manufacturing-vs-3d-printing/#:~:text=3d%20printing%20is%20a%20computer,down%20

successive%20layers%20of%20materials.&text=Whereas%2C%20traditional%20manufacturing%20

involves%20high%20cost%20of%20manufacturing%20and%20shipping.

Redwood, B. (n.d.). 3D printing low-run injection molds. 3D HUBS. https://www.3dhubs.com/knowledge-
base/3d-printing-low-run-injection-molds/#introduction

Remuzzi, A., & Remuzzi, G. (2020). COVID-19 and Italy: What next? The Lancet, 395(10231), 1225–1228.
https://doi.org/10.1016/S0140-6736(20)30627-9

Rezai, P., Wu, W.-I., & Selvaganapathy, P. R. (2012). 1—Microfabrication of polymers for bioMEMS. In S.
Bhansali & A. Vasudev (Eds.), MEMS for Biomedical Applications (pp. 3–45). Woodhead Publishing.
https://doi.org/10.1533/9780857096272.1.3

Rhodes, M. (2015, January 8). A Brilliantly Designed Hazmat Suit for Ebola Workers. Wired. https://www.
wired.com/2015/01/brilliantly-designed-hazmat-suit-ebola-workers/

Rubin, R., Abbasi, J., & Voelker, R. (2020). Latin America and Its Global Partners Toil to Procure Medical
Supplies as COVID-19 Pushes the Region to Its Limit. JAMA, 324(3), 217–219. https://doi.org/10.1001/
jama.2020.11182

Safety & Health Practitioner (SHP). (2015, October 1). PPE: Hazmat suits – your complete buyer's guide. https://
www.shponline.co.uk/procurement-guides/hazmat-suits-your-complete-buyers-guide/

Santa Clara University Engineering Design Center. (n.d.). Injection Molding Overview. http://www.dc.engr.
scu.edu/cmdoc/dg_doc/develop/process/molding/b2500001.htm

Sarda, P. (2020, April 29). India's PPE crisis puts workers in the line of fire. Forbes India. https://www.
forbesindia.com/article/coronavirus/indias-ppe-crisis-puts-workers-in-the-line-of-fire/59073/1

Saul, H. (2014, October 17). Hazmat suits: What are they and how do they protect medics against ebola?
Independent. https://www.independent.co.uk/life-style/health-and-families/ebola-outbreak-what-is-a-
hazmat-suit-9802377.html

Scalzaretto, N. (2020, March 31). 3D printing initatives to provide PPE equipment for hospitals. The Brailian
Report. https://brazilian.report/tech/2020/03/31/3d-printing-initiatives-ppe-equipment-brazilian-
hospitals/

Schwartz, J., King, C.-C., & Yen, M.-Y. (2020). Protecting Healthcare Workers During the Coronavirus Disease
2019 (COVID-19) Outbreak: Lessons From Taiwan's Severe Acute Respiratory Syndrome Response.
Clinical Infectious Diseases, 71(15), 858–860. https://doi.org/10.1093/cid/ciaa255

Seeger, A. (2011, July 25). Collecting Celluloid, the First Semi-Synthetic Plastic. The Atlantic. https://
www.theatlantic.com/technology/archive/2011/07/collecting-celluloid-the-first-semi-synthetic-
plastic/242423/

Shieber, J. (2020, April 6). Apple has sourced over 20 million protective masks, now building and shipping face shields. TechCrunch. https://techcrunch.com/2020/04/05/apple-has-sourced-over-20-million-protective-masks-now-building-and-shipping-face-shields/.

Shukman, D. (2020, May 31). Coronavirus: The mystery of asymptomatic 'silent spreaders'. BBC. https://www.bbc.com/news/uk-52840763

Simplify3D. (2020, April 15). Lessons From the Field – 3D Printed Face Shields. https://www.simplify3d.com/lessons-from-the-field-3d-printing-face-shields/

Sink, J. (2020, May 19). President Trump Says America's 1.5 Million Coronavirus Cases Are 'Badge of Honor' for Testing. Time. https://time.com/5839262/trump-badge-of-honor-coronavirus/

Skrzypczak, N. G., Tanikella, N. G., & Pearce, J. M. (2020). Open Source High-Temperature RepRap for 3-D Printing Heat-Sterilizable PPE and Other Applications [Preprint]. ENGINEERING. https://doi.org/10.20944/preprints202005.0479.v1

Slant 3D. (2020). The Problems with 3D Printed Respirator Masks https://www.slant3d.com/slant3d-blog/the-problems-with-3d-printed-respirator-masks.

Statt, N. (2020, May 25). 3D printers are on the front lines of the COVID-19 pandemic. The Verge. https://www.theverge.com/2020/5/25/21264243/face-shields-diy-ppe-3d-printing-coronavirus-covid-maker-response.

Styles, G. (2018, March 15). 3D Printing Not Yet Ready to Disrupt Plastic Injection Molding. Machine Design. https://www.machinedesign.com/3d-printing-cad/article/21836513/3d-printing-not-yet-ready-to-disrupt-plastic-injection-molding

Swennen, G. R. J., Pottel, L., & Haers, P. E. (2020). Custom-made 3D-printed face masks in case of pandemic crisis situations with a lack of commercially available FFP2/3 masks. International Journal of Oral and Maxillofacial Surgery, 49(5), 673–677. https://doi.org/10.1016/j.ijom.2020.03.015

Tabary, M., Araghi, F., Nasiri, S. & Dadkhahfar, S. (2020, May 8). Dealing with skin reactions to gloves during the COVID-19 pandemic. Infection Control & Hospital Epidemiology, 2020, 1–2. https://doi.org/10.1017/ice.2020.212

Tarfaoui, M., Nachtane, M., Goda, I., Qureshi, Y., & Benyahia, H. (2020). 3D Printing to Support the Shortage in Personal Protective Equipment Caused by COVID-19 Pandemic. Materials, 13(15), 3339. https://doi.org/10.3390/ma13153339

Tétrault, M. (2020, April 15). Health Canada Responds to COVID-19: Here's What You Need to Know About its Expedited Approval Processes. Global Legal Group. https://iclg.com/briefing/13460-health-canada-responds-to-covid-19-here-s-what-you-need-to-know-about-its-expedited-approval-processes

The Canadian Press. (2020, April 03). Trump orders 3M to stop sending N95 masks to Canada. OHS Canada Magazine. https://www.ohscanada.com/breaking-trump-orders-3m-stop-sending-n95-masks-canada/

The Economist (2011, February 10). Print me a Stradivarius. https://www.economist.com/leaders/2011/02/10/print-me-a-stradivarius

Thomasnet. (2020). How to Make Face Shields for Coronavirus/COVID-19. https://www.thomasnet.com/articles/plant-facility-equipment/how-to-make-face-shields-for-coronavirus-covid-19/

Thomas Engineering Company. (2015, June 26). A Brief History of Metal Stamping. http://www.thomasengineering.com/blog/a-brief-history-of-metal-stamping/#:~:text=The%20first%20attempts%20at%20the,is%20now%20modern%2Dday%20Turkey.

Thomas Industry. (n.d.). Top Hazmat Suit Manufacturers and Suppliers. https://www.thomasnet.com/articles/top-suppliers/hazmat-suit-manufacturers-and-suppliers/

Thomas Industry. (2020). How to Make Medical Gloves for Coronavirus/COVID-19. https://www.thomasnet.com/articles/other/how-to-make-medical-gloves/

Thompson, N. (2020, April 26). Coronavirus: Volunteers use 3D printers to produce PPE amid outbreak. Global News. https://globalnews.ca/news/6870488/coronavirus-3d-print-ppe/

Tino, R., Moore, R., Antoline, S., Ravi, P., Wake, N., Ionita, C. N., Morris, J. M., Decker, S. J., Sheikh, A., Rybicki, F. J. & Chepelev, L. L. (2020, April 27). COVID-19 and the role of 3D printing in medicine. 3D Printing in Medicine, 6(1), 11, s41205-020-00064–00067. https://doi.org/10.1186/s41205-020-00064-7

Tomazin, F. (2020, April 5). Ahead of the curve: five other countries winning the battle against coronavirus. The Sydney Morning Herald. https://www.smh.com.au/world/asia/ahead-of-the-curve-five-other-nations-winning-the-battle-against-coronavirus-20200424-p54my1.html

Topping, A. (2020, April 24). Sexism on the Covid-19 frontline: 'PPE is made for a 6ft 3in rugby player'. The Guardian. https://www.theguardian.com/world/2020/apr/24/sexism-on-the-covid-19-frontline-ppe-is-made-for-a-6ft-3in-rugby-player

United Nations Economic Commission for Latin America and the Caribbean (UNECLAC) (2020, May). Restrictions on the export of medical products hamper efforts to contain coronavirus disease (COVID-19) in Latin America and the Caribbean. https://www.cepal.org/en/publications/45511-restrictions-export-medical-products-hamper-efforts-contain-coronavirus-disease

United Nations Information Centres Rio (UNIC Rio). (2020). Brazilian artisans make protective gear to protect against COVID-19 https://www.un.org/en/coronavirus/brazilian-artisans-make-masks-protect-against-covid-19

University of California, Merced. (n.d.). Types of PPE. https://ehs.ucmerced.edu/researchers-labs/ppe/selection

U.S. Food and Drug Administration (FDA). (2020a). 3D Printing in FDA's Rapid Response to COVID-19. https://www.fda.gov/emergency-preparedness-and-response/coronavirus-disease-2019-covid-19/3d-printing-fdas-rapid-response-covid-19

U.S. Food & Drug Administration (FDA) (2020b). Medical Gloves for COVID-19. https://www.fda.gov/medical-devices/coronavirus-covid-19-and-medical-devices/medical-gloves-covid-19#shortages

U.S. Food and Drug Administration (FDA). (2020c). N95 Respirators, Surgical Masks, and Face Masks. https://www.fda.gov/medical-devices/personal-protective-equipment-infection-control/n95-respirators-surgical-masks-and-face-masks#:~:text=An%20N95%20respirator%20is%20a,around%20the%20nose%20and%20mouth.

U.S. Food and Drug Administration (FDA). (2020d, April 5). 3D Printing of Medical Devices and Accessories during COVID-19. https://www.fda.gov/medical-devices/3d-printing-medical-devices/faqs-3d-printing-medical-devices-accessories-components-and-parts-during-covid-19-pandemic.

Ventola, C. L. (2014, October). Medical Applications for 3D Printing: Current and Projected Uses. Pharmacy & Therapeutics, 39(10), 704–711. https://www.ncbi.nlm.nih.gov/pmc/articles/PMC4189697/

von Übel, M. (2019, July 13). The 3D Printing Materials Guide. All3DP. https://all3dp.com/1/3d-printing-materials-guide-3d-printer-material/

Vordos, N., Gkika, D. A., Maliaris, G., Tilkeridis, K. E., Antoniou, A., Bandekas, D. V., & Ch. Mitropoulos, A. (2020). How 3D printing and social media tackles the PPE shortage during Covid – 19 pandemic. Safety Science, 130, 104870. https://doi.org/10.1016/j.ssci.2020.104870

Walsh, N. P., Shelley, J., Fortuna, R., & Bonnett, W. (2020, June 13). Nurse leader accuses Brazil of sacrificing medics to coronavirus. CNN. https://www.cnn.com/2020/06/12/americas/brazil-coronavirus-nurses-doctors-crisis/index.html

Wan, W. (2020, July 8). America is running short on masks, gowns and gloves. Again. The Washington Post. https://www.washingtonpost.com/health/2020/07/08/ppe-shortage-masks-gloves-gowns

Watson, K. & Silva, V. (2020, April 12). Why coronavirus could be catastrophic for Venezuela. BBC News. https://www.bbc.com/news/world-latin-america-52204225

Weir, F. (2020, June 9). Coronavirus shortages give Russia's charity sector a new spark. The Christian Science Monitor. https://www.csmonitor.com/World/Europe/2020/0609/Coronavirus-shortages-give-Russia-s-charity-sector-a-new-spark

Wesemann, C., Pieralli, S., Fretwurst, T., Nold, J., Nelson, K., Schmelzeisen, R., Hellwig, E., & Spies, B. C. (2020). 3-D Printed Protective Equipment during COVID-19 Pandemic. Materials, 13(8), 1997. https://doi.org/10.3390/ma13081997

Whalen, J., Morris, L., Hamburger, T., & McCoy, T. (2020, April 4). White House scrambles to scoop up medical supplies worldwide, angering Canada, Germany. The Washington Post. https://www.washingtonpost.com/business/2020/04/03/white-house-scrambles-scoop-up-medical-supplies-angering-canada-germany/

White, J. L. (1999). Fifth of a Series: Pioneer of Polymer Processing John Wesley Hyatt (1837–1920).

International Polymer Processing, 14(4), 314–314. https://doi.org/10.3139/217.9904

Wilkinson, S. (2020, April 30). PPE Doesn't Fit Women & It's Putting Them At Risk. Refinery29. https://www.refinery29.com/en-us/2020/04/9760085/women-ppe-mask-one-size-fit-risk-covid

Willsher, K., Borger, J., & Holmes, O. (2020, April 4). US accused of 'modern piracy' after diversion of masks meant for Europe. The Guardian. https://www.theguardian.com/world/2020/apr/03/mask-wars-coronavirus-outbidding-demand

Worby, C. J., & Chang, H.-H. (2020). Face mask use in the general population and optimal resource allocation during the COVID-19 pandemic. Nature Communications, 11(1), 4049. https://doi.org/10.1038/s41467-020-17922-x

World Health Organization (WHO). (2020a). Coronavirus disease (COVID-19) advice for the public: Mythbusters https://www.who.int/emergencies/diseases/novel-coronavirus-2019/advice-for-public/myth-busters.

World Health Organization (WHO). (2020b). Naming the coronavirus disease (COVID-19) and the virus that causes it. https://www.who.int/emergencies/diseases/novel-coronavirus-2019/technical-guidance/naming-the-coronavirus-disease-(covid-2019)-and-the-virus-that-causes-it

World Health Organization (WHO). (2020c, March 3). Shortage of personal protective equipment endangering health workers worldwide. https://www.who.int/news-room/detail/03-03-2020-shortage-of-personal-protective-equipment-endangering-health-workers-worldwide

World Health Organization (WHO). (2020d, March 6). Coronavirus disease 2019 (COVID-19) Situation Report – 46. https://www.who.int/docs/default-source/coronaviruse/situation-reports/20200306-sitrep-46-covid-19.pdf?sfvrsn=96b04adf_4

World Health Organization (WHO). (2020e, March 29). Modes of transmission of virus causing COVID-19: implications for IPC precaution recommendations. https://www.who.int/news-room/commentaries/detail/modes-of-transmission-of-virus-causing-covid-19-implications-for-ipc-precaution-recommendations

World Health Organization (WHO). (2020f, April 2). Coronavirus disease 2019 (COVID-19): Situation Report – 73. https://www.who.int/docs/default-source/coronaviruse/situation-reports/20200402-sitrep-73-covid-19.pdf?sfvrsn=5ae25bc7_6

World Health Organization (WHO). (2020g, April 27). Archived: WHO Timeline - COVID-19. https://www.who.int/news-room/detail/27-04-2020-who-timeline---covid-19

World Health Organization (WHO). (2020h, July 9). Transmission of SARS-CoV-2: implications for infection prevention precautions. https://www.who.int/news-room/commentaries/detail/transmission-of-sars-cov-2-implications-for-infection-prevention-precautions

World Health Organization (WHO). (2020i, July 24). COVID-19 situation in the WHO European Region.

https://who.maps.arcgis.com/apps/opsdashboard/index.html#/ead3c6475654481ca51c248d52ab9c61

World Health Organization (WHO). (2020j, July 24). WHO Coronavirus Disease (COVID-19) Dashboard. https://covid19.who.int/

Yale School of Nursing (YSN) (2020, July 15). From Engineering to Nursing, Cisco Partnership Yields Face Shields. https://nursing.yale.edu/news/engineering-nursing-cisco-partnership-yields-face-shields

Yang, C., Tian, X., Liu, T., Cao, Y., & Li, D. (2017). 3D printing for continuous fiber reinforced thermoplastic composites: Mechanism and performance. Rapid Prototyping Journal, 23(1), 209–215. https://doi.org/10.1108/RPJ-08-2015-0098

Young, L. (2020, July 15). 2 hairstylists with COVID-19 saw 139 clients. Here's why no one caught the virus. Global News. https://globalnews.ca/news/7179530/hairstylist-mask-coronavirus/

Zakaib, G., Wakulowsky, L., Boyd, K. & Vila, E. C. (2020, April 6). 3D printing during COVID-19. Borden Ladner Gervais LLP. https://www.blg.com/en/insights/2020/04/3d-printing-during-covid-19

Zhu, Z., Xu, S., Wang, H., Liu, Z., Wu, J., Li, G., Miao, J., Zhang, C., Yang, Y., Sun, W., Zhu, S., Fan, Y., Hu, J., Liu, J., & Wang, W. (2020). COVID-19 in Wuhan: Immediate Psychological Impact on 5062 Health Workers [Preprint]. Psychiatry and Clinical Psychology. https://doi.org/10.1101/2020.02.20.20025338